TWO HANDS

The Gamechanger Guide *for* Manual Therapists

Dr WAEL MAHMOUD
Osteopath & Acupuncturist

Dedication

Mum, Dad, Louise, Grace, Amina & Adam.

There are, of course, no words that are enough to express the individual and unique contributions you've each made to this book. How ironic.

© Wael Mahmoud 2021

All rights reserved. No part of this publication may be reproduced, stored in a retrieval system, or transmitted in any way or by any means, electronic, mechanical, photocopying, recording or otherwise, without the prior written permission of the author.

Design & Typesetting: Leigh Ashforth – watershed design, Melbourne
Cover Photograph: iStock.com/Atstock Productions, Khet Bangna, Thailand

Contents

Testimonials v
Introduction vi

Going solo	1	Thinking on paper	73
Changing course	8	You're in sales	76
Class 101	10	Selling feelings	77
Sharp and crisp	13	All ears	79
Infinite opportunities	15	Finding gold	81
Who will eat your cake?	16	Two-way street	86
Outliers	18	Lifelong partners	87
How not to fit in	21	Systems and processes	88
Where do you live?	25	First contact	89
Differentiators	27	Your greatest asset	94
Disrupters	30	Engage early	98
Deus Ex Machina	33	Opening ceremony	100
Pareto Principle	36	Body language	103
Looking in from the outside	42	Perfect practice	104
Apprenticeship	43	Ready?	106
Pie in the sky	48	Who's in charge?	108
Don't hold on too tight	51	A rod for your own back	109
Learning to fish	54	Opening line	110
Head start	55	What happened next?	113
My teachers, mentors and resilience	59	The shepherd and the flock	116
		Matching	119
'Plane' sailing – not	65	Think ahead	120

Who do you know?	124
Starting at the end	126
The finale	128
We, not I	129
A right to know	133
Listen more than you speak	134
Contested two	136
Don't do this!	138
Long John Silver	148
Consent	150
King of the castle	151
Be curious	154

It's a numbers game	157
Agree to disagree	161
Hiring and firing	163
Imaginary rules	170
"The best yes is to say no"	174
Borrowing from others	177
How much are you worth?	182
Set and forget	185
What next?	190
Dedication	*193*
About the author	*194*

Testimonials

❝ *Two Hands* provides fascinating insights and practical advice from someone with over 30 years of professional experience in the healthcare industry. Highly recommended for all healthcare practitioners. ❞

Jarrod Vos – Physiotherapist

❝ As a Sports Therapist for the past five years and clinic business owner, I found *Two Hands* highly relatable and thought-provoking: it's an essential guide for any manual therapist. This excellent resource will help students and new grads get ahead of their colleagues by taking meaningful steps with minimal detours along the way. ❞

Sophie Soleman – Sports Therapist – Business Owner

❝ The successful transition from a student at university to a practitioner in private practice, in part, will be dependent upon the quality of mentoring one is provided. *Two Hands* provides a 360-degree mentoring journey – brilliant, candid insights from Wael's extensive clinical, business, and life experiences. The joy of helping people live better lives through improved health cuts through in each chapter - a must-read! ❞

Dr Dian Parry – Osteopath – Clinical Educator
RMIT University & Victoria University

Introduction

Whether you're a final-year student, a new grad or an experienced therapist, I will explain how to find your ideal patients or clients, show you what you can learn from disrupters in the healthcare world and those in other industries, the value of mentoring your team and developing an internship program, why and how to create your social media profile, how to use technology to streamline your business processes and amaze your customers, the do's and don'ts in your treatment room, which KPIs to keep and which to ditch, help you decide on your professional fees and develop your critical value proposition.

Dr Wael Mahmoud, D.O., MAppSci (Acupuncture)
Osteopath & Acupuncturist

Going solo

IN THE END, YOU'RE ON YOUR OWN. This well-used truism describes the hermetic career of a manual therapist. No, really, you're on your own. You're on your own from the start of your career until the day you retire. Your clinic workdays are punctuated by the synchronised arrival and departure of the patients you treat. The arrival of a patient doubles your room occupancy; their departure restores the status quo.

Day 1 usually starts something like this:

> Welcome to the clinic. This is your room and this one's mine. The toilets are down the hall. I might not see you when you leave, so make sure you lock the front door behind you.

As qualified, experienced therapists, we are complicit in a faulty system that does nothing to support or nurture the new graduate. We've taken the new graduate on a long car journey to the middle of nowhere and left them there, standing all by themselves, hoping that they'll find their way to where we are, without a map, a compass, or a plan.

As new and inexperienced stock is added to our respective manual therapy flocks, our professions inevitably become diluted year after year. Instead of embracing each and every one of these precious seeds, feeding and watering them with our experience and knowledge, watching them grow strong and confident, we play a collective roulette game with their careers. The determinator of their career success or failure is chance rather than process, which leads to predictably poor outcomes and disappointment all round.

How did we get here? Well, the training and educational establishments have done their jobs: they've met their brief, ticked all the boxes, met all the requirements that were demanded of them by the professions' boards, government departments, regulatory bodies, and the numerous stakeholders within the hierarchy of the training organisation.

The 'product' has been manufactured as per the 'required' specifications, but the inevitable commodity is fragile and labelled with a short expiry date. If the new graduate isn't cared for and protected from the real world, their vulnerability is exposed; over time, they become a poor reflection of the system that created them. The small step from student to therapist becomes a giant leap of faith.

I am deeply saddened by the many stories I hear from young people who have been let down by the system, new graduates who have worked hard to get into a course, have done all that was asked of them, no matter how irrelevant it seemed. For many, disillusion and frustration start while they are still studying, as they begin to realise that this isn't really what they signed up for. If we look at this experience from a purely transactional perspective, where the customer is the undergraduate student and the manual therapy industry is the vendor, by any metric, the sale fell through or at the very least, serious questions must be asked of the customer service department.

> This course is not evidence-based enough.

> I am more interested in sports rehab than treating the general public.

> My arms are sore already.

> I don't feel confident that I can get a job with the skills I've learnt.

> My friends who are new grads aren't that busy in the clinics they work in.

> I might have to keep my part-time job until I can earn a decent income.

> I earn more money working as a barista than I do as a manual therapist.

Many students drop out during their manual therapy training, opting to do something completely different. A manual therapy course is often the experience that confirms that they've made the wrong choice: manual therapy is not for me.

One could argue, what did you expect? Who really knows what they want to do when they leave school? Maybe a few do, but the majority don't. By contrast, mature-aged students who join the same manual therapy courses as their younger counterparts usually know precisely what they want. They've made a conscious decision to change careers, perhaps starting their first in the healthcare field. They're the ones that sit at the front of the lecture hall, soaking up every ounce of value from their investment. Of course, they would. These mature-age students have reached their decision after completing their apprenticeship in real life, not school.

Of course, that's not to say that only mature-aged students know what they want as a career path. I've met some highly driven and passionate young people who knew their calling while they were still at school. They usually resolve to follow a career in health care after a therapist helped them recover from an injury or accident.

I will never forget the first cohort of Osteopathy undergraduates that I taught at what was then called Phillip Institute of Technology in Melbourne. The year was 1987. This group of students was, and still are, exceptional; they were part of a unique and extraordinary fellowship that spawned new life into a tiny profession compared to Physiotherapy and Chiropractic in Australia. This inaugural group would be the first graduates of a government-funded Osteopathy course in the world. Every one of the fifteen, mostly mature-aged students had a story to tell. I remember them all because most had already accomplished great things before choosing to study Osteopathy.

The first-class osteopaths, as they were subsequently called, began their adult lives in other professions, areas of study and occupations, including nursing, journalism, naturopathy, teaching, biology, science, driving a taxi, a mother of four boys, and even working on a prawn trawler!

As a young man myself at the time, I was continually humbled by their determination, hunger, passion and thirst for knowledge, mainly because their future was largely unknown, given the small size of the profession at the time. Their future success was primarily due to the tireless work of many in the profession, well before their course had even started. The pioneers of this fledgeling profession developed the five-year Osteopathy undergraduate training program against the odds. They laid the groundwork and welcomed the faithful inaugural group with great pride at the finishing line. Things are different now. That finishing line no longer exists for a manual therapy graduate.

Unless you've been around the block a few times and sustained a few knocks along the way, you have no choice but to play the game of chance and hope for the best once you graduate. It's an expensive game to play if you end up losing all the time, money, dreams, hopes and aspirations that you've invested in.

Experienced and established therapists should ask themselves: Is this the best we can do to look after the next generation of therapists, those fresh from the factory, the same factory that created you, all those years ago? New graduates who are hungry for their turn and will eventually be our replacements? Surely, we owe them much more than this pitiful and embarrassing introduction to our respective tribes. As a collective of healthcare professionals, we are sadly setting ourselves up for failure.

If the *Physiotherapy Workforce Report* (July 2016) is anything to go by, we should be very worried. The report, which was authorised and published by the Victorian Government in Australia provides an overview of the physiotherapy workforce in 2015–16. It is based on survey responses from 1037 individual physiotherapists and concludes:

> As with other Allied Health professions, there has been a rapid growth in new graduates entering the physiotherapy profession, but they lack adequate support, with many graduates unable to access positions, particularly in the public sector.
>
> Yet, there is still evidence that the community need for physiotherapy is not being met. While physiotherapists are, on the whole, satisfied with the role they play in improving patient outcomes, they have many underlying grievances that affect retention. These include a lack of clinical pathways,

inequities with medical professions, poor remuneration and a lack of professional recognition. "

The report identifies some key areas of concern that contribute to poor retention rates within the profession, including unrealistic expectations placed upon new graduates, resistance to change by organisations, and poor career development.

One respondent quoted in the report states:

> The biggest problem is the retention of junior physiotherapy staff, and I feel this is a reflection on the university course content and perception of the physiotherapy role not always aligning with the reality of the working environment and scope of practice. "

The attrition rate is alarming within the physiotherapy profession. A staggering 27 per cent of the profession intended to leave within the five years following the report's publishing in 2016. Compared to other allied health professions, such as speech pathology and sonography, the attrition rates for physiotherapy are much higher.

Physiotherapy is not alone. Osteopathy and chiropractic are similar to physiotherapy with respect to practice settings. In a study, 'A snap-shot of attrition from the osteopathy profession in Australia', published in the *International Journal of Osteopathic Medicine* (2016), the authors concluded:

> The most commonly selected reasons for leaving the profession included financial dissatisfaction, family commitments, dissatisfaction/boredom with osteopathic practice, and injury. "

Two of the respondents in the same study indicated that they felt 'isolated' in practice. Furthermore, it's possible that respondents' professional expectations were not met, they received little or no mentoring, or they were not equipped with the skills necessary to be successful in practice.

According to a January 2018 report from the Bureau of Labor Statistics (USA), the average person changes jobs ten to fifteen times (with an average of twelve job changes) during his or her career. Many workers spend five years or less in every job, devoting time and energy transitioning from one to another.

Not that long ago, a healthcare career was considered to be immune from the global trend to flit from one job to another: the healthcare professional chooses a vocation, not a job, a vocation that requires dedication and a passion for helping others; health care is a lifelong passion, not for the dilettante. That was the perception when I started my training in 1981, but the allied health world has been slowly imploding over the last three decades.

The article 'Experienced practitioners' beliefs utilised to create a successful massage therapist conceptual model: A qualitative investigation', published in the *International Journal of Therapeutic Massage and Bodywork* (2017) states that the massage therapy profession has grown exponentially in the United States (USA) over the past twenty-five years, and 35 per cent of massage therapists have been in practice for three years or less. This statistic highlights the massive turnover within the massage therapy profession.

Massage therapy is often a second career, according to the authors of this paper. One may therefore hypothesise that it's a career choice based on prior life experiences and deductions made along the way, not one made in the naive teens after the compulsory consultation with the high school careers advisor. Unfortunately, not many stay along for the ride, less than 43 per cent of US massage therapists have been in practice for more than seven years.

The paper's authors explored what makes a successful massage therapist by interviewing 'successful' massage therapists who have had a minimum of five years of experience. Their findings not only shed light on the uniform themes that are thought to determine success by massage therapists but, by deduction, allow us to reflect on why massage therapists find this vocation so challenging.

Participants explained that it was essential to establish a therapeutic relationship with clients, which required excellent communication skills. No surprises there. "The participants also noted the necessity of understanding business on all levels and the necessity of massage therapists to make business decisions."

Stamina is another critical requirement for success.

One respondent explained:

> Stamina means I can do multiple sessions without it being negatively damaging. It can also be emotional, and physical stamina can be built. The clinical experience will also help create stamina. Stamina will also help you to stay in the profession.

Participants also stressed that learning didn't finish after their initial training but must be continued throughout their careers to build an area of expertise.

Our futures as manual therapists are at stake. We have some problems, but there are many more solutions. We need to do better; in fact, we have an obligation to do better if manual therapy is to survive rather than suffer the consequences of progressive dilution, a dilution in our numbers and the quality of our manual skills which are passed on from one generation to the other.

Changing course

IN THIS BOOK I WILL SHARE EVERYTHING I HAVE LEARNT over the past thirty-five years as an osteopath, acupuncturist, company director, university lecturer and business owner. My greatest teachers are my peers and my patients. They have sharpened the blunt and raw skills that I was taught during my training. They have shaped and focused my mind, but above all, they constantly reminded me what it means to be a manual therapist.

Every patient treatment I've given has been an opportunity to learn, refine, discard, practise, test and re-test. In my case, there have been more than 80,000 of these opportunities to populate my experience database. The larger the database, the better the algorithm. The better the algorithm, the better the outcome, for both practitioner and client.

Nothing gives me more pleasure than knowing that I've treated generations within a family. They've been a part of my life and, in many cases, I call them friends. The variety of patient personalities, ages, professions, sporting backgrounds and human stories has enriched my experience as a therapist and as a person.

My apprenticeship has spanned almost four decades. During this time, I have honed my soft and hard technical skills. By far the greatest lessons that I have learnt are described by job recruiters and human resource managers as 'soft skills'. Soft skills are a cluster of human traits, attributes and qualities that are vital for anyone who deals with people to understand, particularly the people who come to you for help as a therapist. Soft skills underpin the 'hard' technical or mechanical skills that are usually easier to learn and replicate.

I have watched how people in pain or discomfort communicate and behave in our treatment rooms. I understand what patients mean when they use certain words or phrases, present with different postures and facial expressions, and how they describe the location of their pain. I have used this understanding to structure my treatments and my communication with every patient in order to respect their unique presentation at that given moment of our interaction.

I have observed thousands of movement patterns and presentations that I have recorded and interpreted into an extensive knowledge database. This experience has enabled me to unclutter the history taking and examination process so that I can quickly find the key determinants of pain or dysfunction and deliver the right treatment and recovery plan.

This focused simplification process streamlines the infinite number of possible inputs into a funnel, a mature funnel that knows which factors and events to reject and which to accept. Like any complex algorithm, the simplification process must never become static; its strength comes from dynamically responding to new information input and experiences over time.

All good relationships rely on a mutual understanding of expectations, boundaries and trust. The patient–practitioner relationship is no different in that regard. This understanding means that a therapist must not only know what their patients want but, much more importantly, what they don't want or need. Therapists can learn how to build enduring relationships just by understanding how to look and listen for the right cues.

If I achieve one of my goals in writing this book, it will be leaving you in no doubt that you're in business as a healthcare professional. I will draw upon real-life experiences and challenges that I have experienced in my career. I have worked as a contractor in many healthcare businesses, owned and managed my own practices, employed many new and experienced healthcare professionals from different professions, hired business managers, reception staff, virtual assistants both locally and overseas, as well as many other ancillary employees since graduating in 1985.

Each section in this book will provide you with the critical skills, knowledge, processes and advice that I use in my practice and education business every day, and I know they will work for you. I will push you to the edge of your comfort zone, show you how easy it is to become an IT guru and explain why you need to embrace existing and emerging technology now. I will share my reading list with you and tell you what you must never do as a manual therapist and why. I will suggest a list of steps to help you get started as a gamechanger, and help you find the answer to this question: what is my purpose as a manual therapist?

There has never been a better time to stand alone in a space reserved for very few. Now is the time to become extraordinary in a world full of mediocrity. What you must do is find the gaps, dare to venture into open space and avoid the crowds.

Class 101

DID YOUR LECTURERS OR TEACHERS REALLY EQUIP YOU to be a healthcare professional? You might have missed the business for healthcare professionals 101 class at the training institution where you studied, but don't worry, everyone missed it because it doesn't exist.

Your training was heavily skewed towards teaching you how not to stuff up, harm your patient, end your career, or blame the people who trained you. Don't get me wrong, teaching you to be safe is a vital part of your education but so is teaching you how to run a business, make the right decisions and ask the right questions.

This book will help you answer the following crucial business questions and considerations as a manual therapist in the healthcare profession, using real-life experiences, tried and tested systems and processes that I have used successfully in my clinic and education business.

- » Why has there never been a better time to make your unique contribution to the healthcare profession?
- » Who are your ideal patients or clients?
- » What are your extrinsic and intrinsic differentiators?
- » Where can you find the most innovative solutions to your business challenges?
- » What can you learn from disrupters?
- » How can you implement a mentorship program in your business?
- » Why is it important to create your social media profile early?
- » Why is it important to welcome failure as a business owner?
- » How can you find your mentors?

- » What is your product?
- » What are your greatest assets?
- » How can you use technology to grow your business?
- » What is the treatment room vocabulary?
- » How can you build a professional network?
- » Why can cognitive dissonance be fatal?
- » Are KPIs really important?
- » How do I prepare contracts and NDAs?
- » How do I hire and fire people?
- » What is your value proposition?
- » How much should you charge?
- » What is the value of leverage?

The 101-Business Class about how to succeed in the healthcare industry and the do's and don'ts of running a healthcare business are not on the curriculum. The people who taught you the origins and insertions of every muscle in the body, orthopaedic testing, the shoulder joint's biomechanics and the autonomic nervous system pathways are experts. The lecturers at your school are experts in their field, indispensable professionals who know a lot about their chosen academic study interests.

Experts are people who know a lot about very little. This observation is not in any way a criticism of the academics that taught you the fundamental knowledge and skills required for your chosen profession. On the contrary, it's a compliment. If you need to learn something, if you want to learn a skill or gain knowledge about a particular subject, you need to find someone who knows a lot about what you want to learn. You don't want to seek help from someone who knows very little about a lot of things. You definitely don't want to ask for help from someone who claims to know a lot about everything; there are other pejorative names for those people.

So, although your lecturers and teachers are experts in their field, they may not be business experts. After you leave the soft, warm and fuzzy environment of your undergrad training, the sharpness of the real world can seem relatively harsh. There's no safety net anymore. You can't take a history in the student clinic then ask the tutor what to do anymore. Your patients are no longer paying a subsidised fee; they are paying a much higher fee and they want results. There's much more at stake now. However, embracing the challenges that come with the sharp end of private practice has many rewards that extend way beyond your career goals.

Wherever you are in your career, this book will provide you with the missing knowledge and information that you must consider and will enable you to maximise the return on your education investment. The investment in your initial training has been a wise one, with unrivalled and unexpected meaningful rewards.

Sharp and crisp

I STILL REMEMBER MY FIRST DAY at the British School of Osteopathy Student Clinic. I was finally able to observe a real treatment given by a senior student under the supervision of a clinic tutor. My day began with extra attention to the clothes I would wear and the shoes I had bought for this much-anticipated occasion.

My greatest challenge that day was to cycle across London in the crazy busy traffic, with my perfectly ironed, brand new, crisp white clinic tunic in a backpack. I felt many different emotions that morning: excitement, responsibility, pride and, above all, a readiness to begin my professional journey alongside the cohort of my undergraduate year.

As a rookie in this new environment, I acted as though I were a fly on the wall, using my compound vision to absorb, detect, assess, record, and remain invisible, seen but not heard.

Of course, I didn't realise it then, but even now, more than thirty years later, I still experience the exact same feelings every time I walk into my treatment room, especially when I see a new patient. I still feel an overwhelming sense of responsibility juxtaposed against my knowledge and experience, which gives me great confidence that I may be able to help the person before me that day.

Like you, I can help people using nothing more than my two perfectly engineered hands, my eight fingers and, of course, my two remarkable thumbs. We can help alleviate someone's pain just by using what we were born with, the amazing tools at the ends of our arms. This concept still amazes me today. What a privilege and opportunity this is. A gift that very few other professions can boast.

Technology will never replace my sense of touch or feel, at least not in my lifetime or for many generations to come. I have complete autonomy in my treatment room. It's just me and the person I am treating. I decide the how, the what and the when. Everything that happens in the room is up to me. I don't require any special equipment, computer software, machines, gadgets or tools. I don't need anyone to help me. The outcome of every patient's treatment is entirely up to me, good or bad. Few vocations in life afford these freedoms and exceptional rewards.

It has been an absolute honour to have had the opportunity to meet so many wonderful people and try and help them reach their goal, whether that was to eliminate pain, restore mobility, return to work or get back to sport.

One of the great joys of my professional life has been teaching and mentoring hundreds of students and graduates from all the manual therapy professions as part of the intern program I established in my multidisciplinary clinics and now in my role as Director of CPD Health Courses. I love being a therapist, teacher, business owner and mentor.

Now I usually wear an Egyptian cotton collared shirt at work and even when I'm not at work, but that's just me. The crisp white tunic that I used to wear remains a symbol representing my obligation to convey objective clarity in every word I say and every technique I perform. My performance in the treatment room, and it is a performance, must be as crisp as my first clinic tunic.

Infinite opportunities

LIFE PRESENTS ALL OF US WITH INFINITE OPPORTUNITIES.

However, not all of us are granted opportunities to help others in our lives; even fewer of us are afforded the chance to take up a vocation synonymous with trust, respect and responsibility. The healthcare professional is assigned these special rights from the time of graduation and beyond.

Just the mere mention that you are a therapist among new acquaintances invites a degree of genuine interest and curiosity because of the fascination that we all have with our bodies, science and health. We are lucky to have chosen such a rewarding and satisfying career in the healthcare profession. It's one of those rare livelihoods that everyone has a story about and a burning question to ask.

The reason we are all so interested in our bodies and inevitable musculoskeletal dysfunction is a little selfish. We all have a vested interest in either our own medical story or someone else's experiences because our health status profoundly determines our survival, our ability to work and consequently our ability to provide for ourselves and those who might depend upon us. It not only affects us, but it also impacts our family's lives, our relationships and the communities we live in.

Acknowledge and embrace the infinite opportunities to help others as a healthcare professional but never let that turn into hubris.

Who will eat your cake?

IMAGINE THAT ONE DAY one hundred recently qualified pâtissiers each decides to make a cake. The cake represents the culmination of everything they have learnt during their training as a student pâtissier. Each pâtissier is provided with the same ingredients and has access to the same culinary utensils, equipment and cookware. The pâtissiers begin to make their cakes. Like you, they believe they have everything they need at the start of their careers, that each of them has an equal chance of making a fantastic cake.

Despite the apparent level playing field, not all the cakes turn out the same, just like all careers don't turn out the same. Some of the cakes will be too dry, too wet, too soft, too sweet, burnt, overcooked, undercooked and, of course, some will be amazing.

This disparity between the final outcomes of the bake-off is a metaphor for what happens at the start of our careers as healthcare professionals. Our treatment results are hit and miss. We all start out on the same road, but because there's no map and no one guides us in our treatment rooms, we get lost. Not many professions allow their newly hatched offspring to muddle their way to inevitable failure and dissatisfaction between the four walls of a treatment room when the stakes are so high for the customer and the therapist.

Unfortunately, for many manual therapists, this lonely and unsupportive experience is all too common, whether you work in a group practice, or you're the first associate that an experienced practitioner hires, and definitely if you start your career working solo. If you think that your initial training has equipped you with all you need to know, you'd be right; that is, if all you wanted to do was to flatline your way to retirement age, without a whimper.

However, suppose you don't just want to have your head above water, bobbing up and down the inevitable fiscal and treatment result wave pool, never really knowing why others with less training, talent or qualifications seem to be getting ahead. While it seems utterly implausible and counterintuitive that many critical skills and knowledge were not part of your professional and academic curriculum, it is entirely understandable that you will not have noted their omission until now.

By learning and, more importantly, understanding why this missing skill set is so important, you'll generate more referrals, retain more patients, and convert every new patient into a lifelong customer. Every patient or client will, in turn, exponentially increase your experience and confidence. As your experience grows, you will learn how to master your communication skills, using them with every patient to gain their trust and loyalty instantly.

If you are a practice owner and you employ other healthcare professionals, you will be able to confidently support and mentor your team to maximise their true potential and help them achieve successful and rewarding careers.

By understanding the hidden value of teaching, developing and training your reception staff how to maximise every phone call, patient inquiry, face-to-face patient interaction and set up clinical systems and procedures, you will mitigate risk, stay safe, compliant and benefit from rapidly advancing technology which creates enormous efficiencies for your business. Delighting your ideal customer becomes a habit rather than chance.

Outliers

MEDIOCRITY IS NOW THE NORM, not only in the healthcare professions, but in all service industries. As customers, we've had to accept new definitions of previously held beliefs about service expectations. Not that long ago, we used to rate service as either poor, good or excellent. Now we have to quietly acquiesce, surrendering to new rating definitions and scales. All of us must now concede that the old 'poor' is now the new 'good'. The new 'good' has become the best that's on offer, like it or lump it.

We find the new 'good' hard to recognise as 'good' because, after all, we always thought that it was just 'poor', nothing special. As for experiencing the old 'excellent', which is now so rare as to be considered a black swan event for most of us, and if we do ever experience this rare commodity, it will be nostalgic, never tangible, like the good old days. When I say 'the good old days', I don't mean earlier this century; this dramatic insidious reset has happened over the past five to ten years.

Since 2013, I travelled almost every weekend to a different capital city using the same airline. I chose loyalty over price, often paying more for a ticket just to earn more points. The post-COVID world has changed many things that we used to take for granted and there's no doubt that the travel and aviation industries have taken a disproportionate financial hit. Having said that, I'm still shocked by the service experience I've recently endured while flying on the carrier, which I had always believed to be the standard bearer. Everything is now barely average, from the onboard snacks instead of meals, the school dinner offerings in the lounge, to the overly officious ground and inflight staff who, since the COVID-19 pandemic, now enjoy their newfound elevated status and authority. I used to feel special as a regular flyer, but now everyone, regular traveller or not, is just like cattle herded into a feedlot.

Everything changed after the arrival of SARS-CoV-2 in December 2019. The service scale has been no exception. Rather than seizing the once-in-a-lifetime golden opportunity to differentiate themselves from everyone around them, many companies have joined the surrounding herds and formed a homogenous corporate blob. They didn't just snatch defeat from the jaws of victory; they actively ripped it out with everything they could muster in a race to the bottom.

Change cannot be judged as good or bad; it's just change. You must never get bogged down in the details of the change. You can thrive in times of change by quickly accepting the new rules of play, evolving so you are stronger and more resilient than your competitors. This strategy has escaped many of the world's largest companies.

The bar of expectation is so low now that it's barely perceptible. However, this new service scale presents us with tremendous opportunities. We now have the choice to legally implement insider trading. Normally of course, insider trading is an illegal practice that uses information that's not in the public domain to make potentially beneficial trading decisions which may then lead to financial gain. However, right now, you are privy to all the information you need to execute strategies and decisions that will benefit you, your patients, your business and your life by raising the bar.

If you want to rise above mediocrity and you're not interested in sitting comfortably in the middle of the bell curve, in the middle of the flock, you must learn and perfect new skills, mindsets, processes, systems, language, routines, habits and behaviours that will transform you and how you do things. Once this exciting transformation begins, you will realise that there's so much more to what you can achieve in your professional life than merely conforming to the norm. It will be the way *you* do things, and only *you* will do them in this way; it will be your personal signature.

I shall stress this point further to avoid any confusion. The way *you* do things will not be right or wrong, or better or worse; it cannot be judged by anyone but you. Just like a signature, it will be yours to keep. Having your own signature requires you to move away from the comfortable midline of the umbrella-shaped bell curve. You need to risk getting wet by shifting your mindset to the periphery. Inhabitants of the bell curve periphery are known as 'outliers'.

It doesn't matter if you decide to live on the right or the left of the midline, as long as you are on the periphery of the bell curve. What matters is that you've dismissed average, normal, expected and ordinary.

Instead, you've chosen that you want to charge much higher or much lower than the recommended or scheduled fees. Or perhaps you've decided that your ideal customer is the very wealthy or the very poor; it doesn't matter. What matters is not the type of outlier but the fact that you are one, and you embrace the character, actions and behaviours of an outlier in every aspect of your professional life. To be an outlier you need to ignore what the majority believes, says and does. You must adopt the persona of a contrarian. When you see the pack heading in one direction, choose a different path. You'll learn to reject the consensus, take calculated risks, always seek disruption, sense opportunities, then welcome the rewards. When your colleagues ask, "Why?", ask them, "Why not?"

If everyone in your profession is doing something one way and you passively follow, without choosing to ask why, you'll become complicit in your own demise. You'll become one of many, subconsciously conforming and blending into the grey of obscurity. The standardisation process starts during childhood and, if unchecked, it continues perniciously, unchallenged throughout your entire adult life. As this insidious regulatory order continues and invades your professional life, you'll realise that now you have fewer and fewer opportunities to value yourself and your services. You have become an ordinary commodity. Deconstruct the word 'ordinary', and you'll want to run away from it as fast as your legs can carry you. *Ordo* is from the Latin meaning row, series, sequence, rank or just plain dull!

Commodities are products like milk, wheat, gold, and natural gas, which are sold based only on price. Generally speaking, milk is milk, whatever colour carton it's in, and natural gas burns in the same way in every domestic stove. At the end of the day, they all conform as expected without raising any eyebrows. By definition, they're nothing special. Do you want to become known as a commodity? Of course not.

To a healthcare professional, conformity means that it becomes harder for your potential clients to see you among the crowd. It is difficult for you to claim the unique contribution you'd like to make and are certainly capable of offering. Unlike commodities that cannot be discerned from the rare and priceless, you have that choice and ability.

How not to fit in

IT'S SO MUCH EASIER TO BE AN ACOLYTE, ISN'T IT?
After all, heresy was once punishable by execution. Thankfully, the days of the Inquisition are long past, well, in most countries anyway. Even without the threat of execution, no one wants to stand out by wearing the 'wrong' clothes, having a funny name, supporting the wrong team, or even being too clever. Our school system is the very essence of conformity; there's nowhere to hide. Round pegs must find a way to fit into the education model. At the end of your school life, the cookie cutter spits you out as a factory-made square peg, no matter how you started twelve years earlier. You've been conditioned to fit in with your peers and the critical outside world.

When we're talking about business, the problem with fitting in is not just the subsequent lack of differentiation between you and the competition; it's actually much more serious than that. By not differentiating yourself, you've decided not to make a unique contribution using the skills and knowledge you've learnt. You've chosen vanilla as your legacy. Why would anyone choose your vanilla, in a sea of vanilla?

If you put yourself in your customers' shoes, without differentiation, they're left with many variables, which they will consider in choosing you over the other vanilla products on offer. These variables may include your location, opening hours, an online search, proximity to public transport, geography, ease of parking or perhaps your fees.

Some of these variables are mostly out of your control, which leaves your business viability in the precarious realm of risk, chance and probability. Despite the many disadvantages of this approach as a way of ensuring career success, it seems completely logical to, and is widely practised by, most healthcare professionals. The path of the contrarian is undoubtedly counterintuitive to almost all, which is why it's not so well travelled.

Do you really want to look back on your career and realise that the only reason your customers chose you is that your practice was nearer to their work, open late on Thursdays, on their way home, the only one they could afford, or your advert came up first in an online search? Surely not? Many argue that these superficial benefits are decisive variables that must be highlighted and prominently displayed to attract potential sales. I strongly disagree.

List these variables and what you'll have is an admin checklist that every business must complete. You will not win any prizes for completing these mundane prerequisites. You'll just fall at the first hurdle if you don't. None of these checklist items differentiates you from your competition. They merely save you a spot on the starting line. You need to come up with something that's not on the standard checklist.

I remember witnessing an example of a business masterstroke in early 1985 while still in my final year of osteopathy training. A few of my more astute and business-minded student friends placed their clinic's quarter-page adverts in the now irrelevant weighty telephone directory called the Yellow Pages before anyone had even started thinking about where they might set up their clinic, let alone, advertising. The fact that they did this before we had even graduated was a risk worth taking. At that time, this business directory was one of very limited opportunities to advertise your practice, barring expensive weekly or monthly box adverts in the local paper. We have moved on from 1985, so much of what applied then about business rules and advertising doesn't apply anymore.

Although the placement of the advert in the Yellow Pages directory was, in hindsight, a checklist item, the way they jumped ahead of the field was differentiation genius. Not only did their adverts create new leads as soon as they graduated, but their sleepy cohort had to wait a whole year before placing their advert in the Yellow Pages and making their mark.

In the year 2000, Yellow Pages ran a TV advert where the angry boss shouts, "Not happy, Jan" at her personal assistant who is seen fleeing the building because she realises that she's missed the print deadline for that year. So popular was the advert, it became a catchphrase to express discontent. The irony is that if you were to ask any experienced practitioner to rate the potential value of a patient or client who has found them through advertising relative to those they attract through word of mouth, hands down, the latter is the most valuable prospect.

The international bestselling American author, entrepreneur and speaker Seth Godin cleverly summarises the concept of attracting your smallest viable market in this wonderfully simple sentence:

> My product is for people who believe X. I'll focus on people who want Y. I promise that engaging with what I make will help you get Z.
>
> Seth Godin, 2018

By boldly stating that your product or services are just for these types of people and not for every single person who has a muscle or joint injury, you are announcing that you will engage only those true believers. Additionally, you make a promise to help these customers attain what they, and they alone, are looking for. You've defined your customers and arguably, much more importantly, rejected those who will not benefit from your product.

You can't help every single person that presents at your clinic. You cannot perform every technical skill that you learnt during your training in equal measures of competency or efficacy. Not all your customers will like you, agree with you or do what you ask of them. The sooner you accept these facts, reject the ego-mind that tells you that you can be everything to everyone, the faster you'll find your ideal patients and become everything to your followers and raving fans, as Ryan Levesque (2019) refers to them.

TAKE ACTION

Start thinking about your X, Y and Z. To help you get started, ask yourself these simple questions. There are no right or wrong answers but there are some principles you should consider. Always remember that people, including patients of course, don't buy products or services, they buy feelings and experiences. Remember that want and need are two entirely different things. Nobody needs a Shelby Super Car Tuatara, but some people want the fastest road car in the world.

Be granular in your thinking; challenge the first answer that comes to mind. Here are some, hopefully thought-provoking, questions. If we consider your product as your service or the treatment experience you are offering:

- » Who is your product for?
- » What problem does your product solve?
- » What is the story behind your product?
- » Do you believe your story?
- » What do your customers believe?
- » What are the barriers to your story?
- » How will you reach the market for your product?
- » What are the benefits to the customer of buying your product?
- » Why, what and how will your customers tell everyone they know about your product?
- » What are your customer's fears?
- » How will you allay those fears?

Where do you live?

SIXTY-EIGHT PER CENT. This otherwise random ratio represents values within one standard deviation (1SD) of the mean in a normally distributed curve. Most people and, by deduction, most manual therapists live here under the shade of the safest part of the curve, in great comfort and safety.

We've all seen the normally distributed curve on a graph before, the graph used to plot values such as test scores, height, weight, or any other characteristic of a given cohort. The graph's vertical axis, known as the 'Y axis', is on the left side of a page. The horizontal line, called the 'X axis', lies at 90 degrees to the Y axis. Together, the two axes make an 'L' shape.

Plotted on the graph is a symmetrical bell-shaped curved line representing the information we are interested in studying. If we were to draw a vertical line that divides the bell into two halves, splitting the bell into mirror images, that line would be called the centre line and would bisect the X axis at a point equal to the average or mean of the respective data or values we've plotted on the graph.

Your cohort, which includes other skilled manual therapy professionals, has both empirical and theoretical characteristics such as exam results, academic knowledge, manual skill levels, ability to recall critical red flags, and the thought process of clinical reasoning.

Like the last bowl of porridge in the fairy tale Goldilocks and the Three Bears, 68 per cent of therapists feel just right, not too hot nor too cold. In the world of only one standard deviation from the average, you'll enjoy the company of others who like to be able to see the centre line at all times, never straying into less protected terrain or far from the shelter that the middle of the bell curve provides.

Goldilocks was a 68 percenter who enjoyed her standard deviation life. The timeless tale, transformed from its original version by Joseph Cundall (1849), is about a young girl with golden hair who goes for a walk in the forest one day and accidentally stumbles upon the home of three bears.

While the bears were out, she made important choices about which bowl of porridge she would eat from, which chair she would sit on, and which bed she would lie on. She chose average every time. Not too hot, not too cold. Not too big, not too small. Not too hard, not too soft. These low-risk decisions are consistent with the humdrum of a 1SD post code.

While you were a student, you learnt how to perform dozens of valuable technical skills, committed thousands of essential facts to memory, attended hundreds of hours of lectures, and stayed up late on way too many occasions just so you could meet the assignment submission deadline at midnight. You correctly regurgitated the required knowledge during your exams, which means that you can now proudly enjoy looking at the parchment bearing your name and award hanging on your pastel-coloured clinic room wall. Congratulations.

The deceptive security and safety of a 1SD address will inevitably lead to mediocrity, disillusion, staleness, boredom, frustration, resentment and discontent.

Relocation is a consideration at any time during your career, whether your career is newly hatched or many years on. A new residential landscape brings with it a constriction that forces valuable and exciting new opportunities. The extraordinary outcomes that result from a move to the less shaded parts of the bell curve are the antithesis of the consequences of being stuck in the middle of 1SD.

Differentiators

ONE WAY TO THINK ABOUT DIFFERENTIATORS is to group them as either extrinsic or intrinsic. Extrinsic differentiators might include things such as pricing, the type of treatment table you use, the colours included in your branding, your window display, or the copy you use on your website. The beauty of differentiators is that almost any attribute is acceptable. You're in control of how you choose to set yourself apart.

Extrinsic types of differentiators are vulnerable to cloning by your competitors. It's easy for like businesses to copy your well-thought-out pricing strategy, slightly tweak your tag line, and call it their own or match your A-board images because they look great.

This doesn't mean that you should avoid extrinsic differentiators, but you should consider how you can use a mixture of extrinsic and intrinsic differentiators to protect against plagiarism. I'll explain later about the importance of trademarking in order to protect your intellectual property.

Intrinsic differentiators are immune from copying; they're based on you, as a therapist, and your particular skill set, technical know-how, manual craftsmanship, personality and inherent behaviours. No one can copy you exactly. One way to create differences between you and the opposition is to master your craft using intrinsic differentiators. If you develop and refine your treatment skills, diagnostic accuracy, injury rehabilitation programs, expert knowledge base and communication methods, no one can match these or take them away. They're yours to own and keep.

There are many examples of healthcare practitioners who have developed intrinsic skills that are unmatched by their peers. They become the go-to therapist for a particular type of treatment or intervention. The treatment is usually highly specific to a region of the body or uses a specific technical approach. These therapists have narrowed their minimal viable market to patients looking for the one, not the many.

We've all heard our friends and family saying, "You should see Trevor, my back guy; he fixes me every time", or "I wouldn't let anyone touch my neck except for Simone, she's so good. I used to get daily headaches till I saw her, now I never miss my monthly maintenance treatments."

I recall a story about two of my patients who met for the first time on a beautiful 18-hole golf course two hours' drive from my practice one autumn afternoon. One of these men started talking about the degree of freedom he now enjoys after he first visited his back guy a few years ago. He had tried everyone before seeing this one therapist whom his brother had recommended. He explained that he now rarely experiences the disabling back spasms he used to get, which stopped him from playing golf. They used to be bad enough to stop him from even getting out of bed.

At this point in the conversation, the story about his back guy switched from passing conversation to spirited banter between the golfing pair. The other golfer took umbrage at the accolades his playing partner was bestowing on his therapist, and friendly competition about which one of them had the best back guy ensued. Both golfers thought that their guy was better than the other golfer's. Anyone listening to this verbal tussle would be able to testify that the descriptions the two men gave of their respective therapists changed from simply someone who fixes their backs to an almost superhuman magician who could do no wrong and enjoyed a 100 per cent track record of pain relief.

The amusing conversation continued for at least three holes of golf; it may have continued for longer, but then one asked the other to reveal the identity of their heroic therapist. The two men laughed at themselves when they discovered they were both talking about the same therapist. The golfers had created their own stories about their therapist and sincerely believed them to be true. The psychological effect of their treatment experience was feelings of joy, happiness, contentment, pleasure, relief and exhilaration. All these emotions were inextricably connected to their love of the game of golf and their ability to play the game without back pain or limitations to their function.

Although this story contains much hyperbole and exaggeration, I like to use it when mentoring younger associates, not to amplify my abilities or reputation, but to demonstrate the power of a story. Without a doubt, customers' stories can strongly influence their opinions and actions. Better still, these stories spread like a virus. What's the story that you would like your patients or clients to spread about you?

Disrupters

LET'S LOOK AT SOME WELL-KNOWN EXAMPLES of businesses that have defined their product, that know their ideal customer intimately, and how their product will make their perfect customer feel when they buy it.

The Fat Duck is an excellent example of a business based on evoking emotions through the stimulation of all five senses. Everything about this iconic restaurant, including the physical appearance of its British celebrity chef-owner, Heston Blumenthal, is different. Calling the Fat Duck a restaurant is like calling a Ferrari a car. Blumenthal says that his restaurant is not a restaurant. It's an experience from the minute you make your reservation to the minute you leave. Dining at the Fat Duck is a culinary experience that evokes childhood food memories, feelings of excitement, delight, surprise, anticipation and expectation. Unlike any other mundane dining experience, it messes with your mind.

The small fortune that you'll pay at the end of the Fat Duck dining experience is equivalent to the average monthly food bill for a small family. This pragmatic comparison is a little unfair. The two products that we are trying to compare are incomparable. One represents the monetary value of essential foods needed to sustain life in a given month; the other represents an experience lasting a few hours that you don't *need* to stay alive but just *want*. Want and need are entirely different verbs.

You're buying an experience, a story to tell others about, a chance to eat food that engages all five senses simultaneously, one that conjures up memories of childhood treats dressed up as modern culinary representations, and visual replicas of seasonal fruit or everyday vegetables that challenge your brain like an Escher drawing. If you think eating at the Fat Duck is about the food alone, you're missing the point. From the minute the first thought about eating at this three Michelin Star restaurant enters your mind, the journey begins, a trip into fantasy food land that creates an enduring story to share with your family and friends. Blumenthal and his team have created a product that has essential differentiating characteristics from a mere plebeian restaurant. The uncompromising diners who the Fat Duck attracts are the few, not the many; they're focused on the ultimate dining experience. These customers believe in the product and are prepared to wait up to five months just to be granted a coveted table. Like many businesses that know the customers they're after, the Fat Duck experience is symbiotic, two pieces of a jigsaw looking for each other. When they find each other, they lock and become engaged, each knowing they belong together. Many of these businesses don't initially make sense; they're too expensive, too cheap, have too long a waiting list, are too hard to find, too far, too crowded, and the list of rationalisations goes on.

Why is there always a queue outside the Louis Vuitton store in the Avenue des Champs-Élysées in Paris? Why would anyone pay Richard Branson's Space Flight company, Virgin Galactic, $250,000 for a 2.5-hour trip into space? Why do some people buy everyday groceries at Harrods in southwest London when the equivalent products are available at a fraction of the cost in Aldi? Why do foodies and gym junkies use the La Croix bottled mineral water brand, not as necessary hydration but as a status symbol?

All these brands have one thing in common: they've differentiated themselves from the rest. They're different kettles of fish. There are many more we haven't even mentioned, such as Billabong, Supreme, easyJet, Ikea, Dollar Shave Club, Subway, Apple, Hard Yakka, Aldi, Netflix, Airbnb and Anytime Fitness. Although they have all differentiated themselves, they haven't all done this based on the same variables. Differentiation is not about price alone; price comes way down the list of considerations. However, guaranteeing that your product is cheaper than everyone else's, whenever you can, is a compelling differentiator.

When the Greek-Cypriot entrepreneur Stelios Haji-Ioannou founded the low-cost airline easyJet in 1995, his business model was all about making it easy, enjoyable and affordable to travel again and again. The model offered something different and challenged the old guard. Everything about the easyJet brand emphasises the word 'cheap'. Visitors to its site are asked if they're looking for cheap flights because if they are, they've come to the right place. On offer are a large selection of low-cost flights and deals.

easyJet's minimum viable market are air travellers who want to travel as cheaply as possible, frequently and easily as possible; they don't want to use or pay extra for a lounge; they prefer to engage with a company that is going to offer them a 'pay for what you get' experience, rather than force them into paying for food and luggage allowance they don't need or want. Given that easyJet's business model is based on cheap air travel, a viable revenue stream and subsequent profits depend on a high volume of travellers, not price.

Uber is another business that has differentiated itself and disrupted the taxi industry by offering another option to a market of customers attracted to the very subtle differences between conventional taxis and the Uber ride share experience. Uber's differentiation strategy is not based on price, speed of travel, comfort or any apparent variables related to getting from A to B. The Uber customer is attracted by the ability to order a car by pressing a button on an app, rather than having to line up in a traditional taxi rank queue. They don't want to compete with other would-be passengers in a line or hail one by waving and whistling, hoping to catch the driver's attention. We have all seen the ride share customer standing next to a line of empty taxis gleefully choosing an UberX, Comfort or UberXL ride on their phone. They have made a choice based on something other than pure availability.

They want to order it when they're ready, and they want it to come to them. The Uber App gives them the ability to choose where they want to be picked up, gives them an ETA, offers them a choice of cars, asks them whether they prefer conversation or silence, and even tells them how much they'll pay before they click Confirm. The most attractive feature of the Uber offering is the invisible payment method. At the end of the trip, the passenger simply gets out of the car, and the payment is made 'automagically'. This seamless transaction occurs without a word being spoken. There's no need for you to make sure you have enough cash ready or a need to play the guessing game about how much your journey will cost. Even the sometimes-awkward question of how much shall I tip is solved by allowing the passenger to tip the driver after their trip and even compliment their ride experience. These small changes can add massive differentiation to what has previously been accepted as a commodity purchase.

Deus Ex Machina

THERE ARE MANY EXAMPLES OF HEALTHCARE PRACTITIONERS who are clearly differentiating themselves and standing out from the crowd.

Take Marty McCullock, an osteopath who owns a practice in Wollongong, New South Wales, Australia. Marty's clinic is called The Clinic Osteopathy & Dry Needling. His clinic's name clearly explains what is on offer at his business: osteopathy and dry needling. Simple.

Marty and his clinic represent everything that he loves about life. The clinic is Marty's story on show for everyone to see and read. Marty is making a statement about who he is, and who his product is for. His customers leave his business knowing they belong to a tribe. Marty's tribe share the belief that their treatment experience is unique and valuable; it evokes deep emotions of belonging and ownership. How does he achieve this?

If you think about retail businesses in any high street, their windows are the most valuable piece of floor space. The visual merchandising specialists create their brand's look and feel, using every inch of the available display space to punctuate the potential customer's intended course along the footpath, attempting to hook them and divert them into their store. Marty has taken this retail concept to another level, literally another level. You see, Marty loves motorbikes, not all motorbikes though; he's incredibly selective and loyal to a few iconic brands.

Marty has a 1960s Honda Dream 50 Café Racer replica motorbike sitting proudly on a raised ledge on the right side of the front door to his clinic. The thing is that Marty's clinic is not on the ground floor. It took a lot of heaving, pulling, and careful lifting to rest this important piece of Honda motorbike history all the way up two flights of stairs.

The motorbike was specially built to commemorate Soichiro Honda, the founder of the Honda Motor Company, and his racing dreams. It celebrates the company's earliest beginnings in Japan to the multinational conglomerate it is now.

It's no coincidence that Deus Ex Machina, which literally translates as 'A god from a machine', was the company that imported the Honda Racers from Japan into Australia. Deus Ex Machina is a unique brand that is all about differentiation from the masses. It's also no coincidence that Deus Ex Machina is one of Marty's favourite brands.

The word 'favourite' is an understatement here. When I say, 'favourite brand', we need to understand that, for Marty and others like him, Deus is not like wearing a Nike T-shirt or Vans footwear because they're comfortable and the logo looks great with your jeans. No. Deus is much more than just the functionality that the products provide. These products represent an ecclesiastical connection to the icon and a tribal connection between its followers. It's no surprise that Marty's closest friends are also Deus tribesmen.

As patients are dry needled, stretched, manipulated and returned to function on Marty's Athlegen treatment table, they're enjoying listening to an eclectic music library populated by the big hitters, spanning sixty years, starting in the 1920s, including the First Lady of Song, Ella Fitzgerald, Louis (Satchmo) Armstrong, Led Zeppelin, Jimi Hendrix and, arguably the perfect accompaniment to any manual therapy session, Creedence Clearwater Revival's, 'Have You Ever Seen the Rain?'

By now, you won't be surprised to learn that these music legends are heard in their purest form through the delicate but potent contact between stylus and vinyl that rotates at a constant speed on the Marley X Audio Technica turntable positioned next to a pine desk in Marty's treatment room. It would be a crass confliction to listen to these timeless classics through the predictable digital sound of a CD player connected to the default computer speakers of a mundane laptop.

Marty is surrounded by the brands he loves; he's making an unapologetic statement about who he is to his patients and indeed the other therapists and staff he employs. He stands wearing a black Deus Emporium cap, the white short-sleeved cotton Deus Milano Address shirt and, of course, he completes the look by wearing a black rather than medical blue latex-free glove on his non-needling hand. Marty expresses himself through his clothes, his favourite brands, his musical tastes and the environment he works in.

This is a great way to differentiate because Marty has answered the simple question:

> If I'm going to work in this room for at least a third of every day, how do make it somewhere that I'll feel comfortable and happy?

There are some downsides to this differentiation model: ironically, the same features that make it unique also make it vulnerable. If your business is built around you, then without you, there is no business. This argument is hardly compelling – all you need to do is look around at the many successful businesses that are built around individuals, Air Jordan, Ben & Jerry's, David Beckham, Carl Zeiss, Christian Dior, The Hershey Company, Hugo Boss, Johnnie Walker and Tag Heuer. Being *you* can be your business.

Pareto Principle

DR PADDI LUND is a Brisbane dentist who closed his practice doors, 'got rid of' 80 per cent of his existing patients, removed all his advertising outside his business, deleted his phone number from the phone book, replaced his reception desk with a cappuccino machine, and now serves his remaining patients, whom he loves to treat, freshly baked 'dental buns' alongside a cup of tea, served in a bone China cup and saucer.

Dr Lund doesn't fit in at all; he's done his level best not to follow the well-trodden professional medical services route travelled by most of his colleagues. He now loves what he does, makes twice as much income, works only twenty-two hours a week and, most importantly, he's much less stressed.

The stimulus that drove Dr Lund to change who he was working for and serving in his business was how it was making him feel. Work was making him feel miserable. The unhappiness affected his staff, patients, personal life and all those around him. He decided that if he spent the lion's share of his working week in a place of misery, something had to change.

Why on earth would anyone spend irreplaceable time in a place that made them feel less than excited, happy, useful, rewarded and fulfilled every minute of the day? It's almost as though we need to perform work to feel less guilty about play and, worse still, the harder we work, the more we think we deserve a reward.

Dr Lund decided to build a business that makes him happy. What followed this decision was a period of introspection and decisions about what makes him happy or unhappy. Paddi describes how it's a lot easier to just get on with things, even if they don't feel right. People find introspection and reflection quite hard and even quite confronting, given the possible outcomes when looking within. He set about adding all the things to his business that made him happy and taking away the things that didn't. His goal was to make his customers happier than they were before they met him. This was his product. Dentistry was the service he supplied to deliver the product. His purpose in his business was to make people happy.

His approach was also to make himself happy to be able to make others happy. Making his patients happy made him happy. By surrounding himself with happy people, he became happier too. It became a tremendous vicious cycle. As part of his product, everything he would create had to provide happiness or it could not be part of his business.

Paddi realised that people are greatly affected by how other people treat them. This relationship dramatically impinges on our happiness. If people are polite and respectful to us, it tends to make us feel good. If they're not, it doesn't. Generally, people want to be treated with politeness and respect. Paddi discovered this by researching the interactions that people had with each other and which of those interactions made people unhappy.

In almost all situations, he found people were unhappy when others did not treat them with respect, were not polite to them – lack of 'please', 'thank you', lack of a smile, and talking about others behind their back. Together with his staff, he made up a list of acceptable standards for communicating with each other. Initially, there were seven rules or standards on the list that Paddi and his staff attempted to live by while working together in his practice. They were not always successful, but everyone noticed a distinct increase in their happiness levels.

Every evening after work, the staff and Paddi would sit down together and score their happiness levels. Invariably, the things that caused a lower score would be a human interaction that didn't go as planned and someone felt disrespected or not thanked. The rules of engagement were not difficult to understand or complicated processes in any way. One example was that if you want something from another staff member, say 'please'. If you receive something from someone, say 'thank you'. If someone says, 'thank you' to you, you say, 'you're welcome', or 'it was a pleasure'. These are basic manners that most of us were taught by our parents when we were children but, somehow, they've been forgotten by many adults in the workplace.

These rules made a big difference to the happiness levels within Paddi's business team. Not only do they live by these rules, but

Dr Lund wrote a book about what he called 'the courtesy system of rules': *Building the Happiness-Centred Business: Business, Happiness and Money Never Mixed ... Until Now* (2006). The book explains how to build a system within a business that makes people happy with each other.

Although they started the system within the team of staff members, they later introduced the system to their patients and invited them to use it when communicating with the staff and therapists. The proviso was that if a patient thought they might find this new approach challenging to comply with, it would be better to find another dentist.

Eventually, Paddi let go of as much as 80 per cent of his existing patient list over time. He took down the signage outside his clinic and only took on new 'special guests' or privileged customers; this was the new term Paddi used to replace patients. Special guests had to be invited by existing customers, ensuring that more of the same demographic would add to the select few. Gone was the walk-in or the patient who found Paddi in the phone book and needed an appointment right now.

Using a business strategy based on scarcity, for every thousand people, Paddi only wanted one special guest. Each guest was educated about good dental health and steered away from a myopic focus on short-term, solution-based thinking about their health. Instead, special guests were guided towards a new way of thinking that takes a long-term prophylactic approach.

This paradigm shift meant that Dr Lund's pricing was no longer inextricably linked to the 'fix', which may have been a filling or crown, but to more of a comprehensive, broader, planned approach to treatment. Instead of guests asking the price of a filling, they began to dissociate a particular intervention with a specific price or fee.

The smell of medical or dental practice is important. Many people are anxious about, even scared of dentists and pain. The scent of Novocain often greets dental practice patients as they walk through the door. Our sense of smell is deeply connected with our emotions, good and bad. He got rid of the Novocain smell by diverting the air from the operating areas outside rather than into the waiting rooms. He also negated Novocain's effect by starting a dental patisserie, where he baked his 'dental buns'.

This changed the smell of his business, which changed the feelings of fear to more desirable feelings of pleasure. He offered tea to his special guests to break down barriers, make them feel happy and cared for. He didn't just offer tea, he would say, "I'm having a cup of tea. Would you like one?" More people said 'yes' because they felt they weren't a bother.

These are just a few examples of healthcare professionals and businesses outside the healthcare field that have managed to differentiate themselves from the rest of their market. Many might think that these examples are a long bow to draw. After all, who can be bothered to bake dental buns or lift a 156-lb motorbike up two flights of stairs? Of course, you can be bothered. Hopefully, you are beginning to see how these seemingly irrelevant actions, habits, personalities and behaviours help to build a strong narrative about your product and who you want to serve.

I look at these stories and get excited by the opportunities to stand out in an overcrowded market. I love the innovation, entrepreneurship and boldness of these business owners who make statements about who they are, what they stand for and how they clearly state that their product is not for everyone.

You might be forgiven for thinking that this business strategy of attracting only a few rather than the many is risky and would likely lead to inevitable business failure. This assumption would likely fall, with many others, under the banner of logical fallacies.

Aristotle is thought to be the Greek philosopher who first wrote about a natural but nevertheless faulty thinking process called *post hoc* fallacies. The full name of this observation is the Latin *post hoc, ergo propter hoc*, which means, 'after this, therefore because of this'. A quick but relatable *post hoc* clinical example might be that your patient returns after treatment and reports that they are much better. The logical fallacy in this context could be that it is entirely related to the treatment you gave them a week ago. Equally fallacious is the alternative presentation, your patient returns after treatment and reports that they are much worse. In either situation, we easily fall into the trap of correlating an observation, in this case a patient's account, with a cause, our treatment effect. Are we sure that our treatment had a positive or negative impact? We must be more careful in drawing sometimes tenuous and often incorrect conclusions.

The natural but short-sighted assumption about attracting the few rather than many is based on the equally blinkered deduction that if I attract fewer people, that means I will not be busy enough, I will not make any money, and therefore I will go broke very quickly. Nothing could be further from the truth.

You need to open your mind and allow your natural curiosity to dictate rather than our often faulty and restricted assumptive thinking patterns. No one said that by standing out from the crowd, you'd attract fewer people. You need to attract your ideal customers. That doesn't mean fewer people. Your perfect customer could be as few as one or as many as hundreds of thousands of people. It all depends on who your product is for. That's the starting point. Once you know that, then the rest becomes so much easier than aiming everywhere but nowhere.

Even if your product is aimed at fewer people than your competitors, that doesn't mean you'll go broke. The easyJet example under the heading 'Disrupters', shows that the airline's product is aimed at the many who want to pay as little as possible. This model is just as viable as the Gulfstream corporate jet experience aimed at the very few customers who have no concern about price.

As though there are not enough examples of *post hoc* fallacies globally, let alone in manual therapy, let's just add this beauty:

> If I open more hours in a week, offer late weekday appointments and weekends, I'll see more clients, and therefore be successful.

No, this is called desperation and desperation leads to burnout.

I love to look at other industries to see what they are doing that I'm not. When was the last time that you visited an online shopping site? Of course, we've all done this, but have you also noticed what they do to promote scarcity? Let's say that you visit an online store looking for a microwave. The site's geo targeting algorithm analyses your hostname and IP address. The site now knows your approximate location and what type of product you're looking for. After a pre-determined time interval, a small but conspicuous pop-up appears in the bottom left-hand side of your screen, which tells you that another customer from a suburb near you has just bought the same or similar microwave for an unbeatable price. Here's the kicker though, the pop-up also says that there are now only two left in stock. Hurry, or you'll miss out. You are immediately filled with a mixture of two emotions, trust and fear. You think, well, if others are buying from here, I should join them because the product must be ok. That's the trust emotion kicking in. Simultaneously, you have FOMO (fear of missing out) created by the pop-up call to action messaging.

Scarcity is the oldest tool in the book. Use it wisely and carefully. Rather than opening your clinic all day, every day, why not become the late-night, the early morning, the weekend, or the nine-to-five clinic? If your ideal patient cannot come in during the day and enjoys the evening appointment experience, don't confuse them and everyone else by opening up at seven in the morning as well. The message has to be clear: I'm only looking for customers who want to come to see me between 6 pm and 9 pm on weekdays. There's a price for everything. By choosing to work at these times, and these times only, you are creating scarcity. Scarcity attracts higher value. These evening appointments must be offered at a higher price than daytime appointments.

While your ideal clients are booking their online appointments, why not let them know how many appointments are left at the time slot they're looking for while they're choosing? Why not change your pricing structure to reflect demand. Are your Saturday morning appointments the same price as the mid-morning weekday appointments? If more of your patients or clients want the Saturday appointments, this demand must be reflected in the price. Look at the airline, tourism, hospitality and petroleum industries. They will all increase prices when there's higher demand. If you want to fly on a popular route at a time that is in high demand, you'll pay more than you would for the same flight two hours earlier or later.

You don't have to take these ideas and try and copy and paste them in their entirety. I've found that the best way to use these ideas is to pick and choose what you want, depending on who your product or service is for. That must be your first question.

Looking in from the outside

I'M A GREAT BELIEVER IN CONSTANT LEARNING, but not just from anyone and everyone.

I have found that the most productive lessons I have learnt came from places that are as distant from my path as possible, the further, the better.

Any challenges you face as a healthcare practitioner are likely to have been encountered by others in the same field. The solutions that others in your industry have found will be ones that you have perhaps already tried and implemented.

Sometimes the answers will work, but often they draw you into the deadly funnel of orthodoxy. This easy option has you solving problems in precisely the same way as your competitors rather than looking for inspiration from other less constricted disciplines and vocations. Your newfound solution could inadvertently box you into acquiescent conformity rather than the delight and excitement of disruption and discord.

I have found new answers, ideas, innovations and designs to countless challenges. Sometimes, I wasn't even looking for an answer in many unrelated industries, businesses and professions. Keep your eyes and ears open and you will be rewarded with untold opportunities for tackling common problems with unique solutions.

Apprenticeship

CAN AN APPRENTICESHIP MODEL BE APPLIED TO THE ALLIED HEALTH PROFESSION? This tried and tested model may offer new ways to train, support and retain those interested in joining the manual therapy professions.

The sharp end for any allied health professional is undoubtedly the private practice environment. It's an insecure environment where your success as a healthcare professional is measured by your most recent performance and that alone. 'You're only as good as your last treatment' is an adage I've always tried to work by. Your job isn't guaranteed by tenure, contract or the endless supply of clients in the government sector.

I'm a great believer in searching for answers in unusual places, down the less trodden paths. We can gain much information and insight if we look for answers to many of our problems by learning from others who are entirely removed from the challenge at hand. The freshness and clarity of new eyes can be all that it takes to resolve a puzzle. Solving the challenge of attrition and disillusion requires change. Change is not always easy, but it is inevitable, necessary, and always possible if you know where to look.

Other industries and those within them have encountered similar challenges. They've looked for answers and found possibilities. These possibilities are precious pieces of knowledge that may assist us in finding our own resolutions or at least direct us away from the slothful acceptance of tradition, institution and convention. Instead, we must welcome and embrace disruption. We must question and reject old thinking if we are to shape our careers and our chosen professions.

The hopeless inauguration into our respective professions should be and can be so much better. It can be much more relevant, supportive, progressive, valuable and rewarding for the new graduate and their respective professions as a whole.

Contrast this experience with the apprenticeship model and its inherent transfer of skills from one generation to the next, without which our most significant structures, buildings and monuments would never have been built. Indeed, entire civilisations, cultures and societies have been built on the values of shared knowledge, craftsmanship and manual techniques, which were passed on from as early as medieval times to the present day.

> Four thousand years ago, the Babylonian Code of Hammurabi required artisans teach their crafts to youth. The records of Egypt, Greece and Rome from the earliest times reveal that skills were also being passed on in this fashion. When youth of olden days achieved the status of craft workers, they became important members of society.
>
> *Apprenticeship: Past and Present*, 1991

This logical process of an apprenticeship served several essential goals so that valuable skills were not lost. They were passed on from a craftsman to an apprentice throughout the internship. This master and apprentice relationship was enduring and had far more wide-reaching scope than the mere transfer of skills. Another benefit included fellowship, friendship, pride and purpose, which were sealed by the acceptance to a guild or trade after the training. These goals complemented each other beautifully, serving to provide employment and income for the apprentice and opportunity and assistance for the experienced craftsman.

Admission to this fraternity was not the conclusion of learning, but a point along the continuum of an evolutionary education process that starts with an interest and concludes with a durable gift from teacher to student.

One of the most prosperous, stimulating, productive and creative periods in human history was 1400 to 1600 in Florence, Italy. Florentines witnessed and benefited from an intense and vigorous cultural, political, artistic and economic rebirth during this relatively short period, where every field of work, study and training flourished and prospered. There were tremendous advances in all the disciplines, including medicine, mathematics, engineering, science, architecture, literature, and art and crafts.

In his biography of Leonardo da Vinci (2018) Walter Isaacson reports that, in 1472, an astonishing 84 woodcarvers, 83 silk workers, 30 master painters, 44 goldsmiths and jewellery artisans all worked in Florence, which was known as the Athens of the Middle Ages.

During this remarkable period, an artist's training began at an early age, sometimes as young as twelve or fourteen, lasting up to eight years. Each student would work under a master artist; their parents would sign a contract that would detail the arrangements. The young apprentice would be looked after by the master artist, who was obliged to provide their charge with food, accommodation, clothes and even pay.

Like other trades, the art guilds, which represented the apprentices much like unions of today, supported their training by negotiating contracts and helping them to sell their paintings independent from their masters. The term 'masterpiece' is derived from the final requirement for an arts apprentice to present a piece of their work to the guild to demonstrate their proficiency before they could graduate from apprenticeship.

The current pathway for many choosing a job in the automotive, building, electrical, landscaping, hair/beauty, manufacturing, painting, plumbing, welding industries is built on the principles of passing on essential knowledge and skills, graded mentoring, commensurate with experience, payment while learning and the provision of employment. Is this an alternative to the contrasting allied health model of a framework built on none of these principles?

Before you get all bourgeois, precariously perched upon high, looking down on the blue-collar proletariat, you'd do well to temper these initial irrational assumptions and consider whether the skills we are required to learn and the knowledge we must acquire as allied health professionals are not dissimilar to those for a trade.

Imagine you decide to become a physiotherapist, osteopath, chiropractor, massage therapist, podiatrist, or exercise scientist, but instead of the current model you could start an allied health apprenticeship. As part of your training, you partner up with one or more mentors representing your chosen career pathway; they're experienced and trained professionals who are willing to take you on as an apprentice.

Your training consists of on-the-job, hands-on training with your mentor, and online and face-to-face training at a tertiary institution. Given access to the standard theoretical knowledge common to almost all allied health professions, you would study together with other apprentices who will reach differing endpoints and share similar theory prerequisites. You're paid from day one, and your wage increases incrementally with experience. Not only are you paid, but your mentor is paid when you are charged out. After an agreed period of time, you can use your newly learnt manual skills, passed on by your mentor and the theoretical knowledge learnt at your college to treat simple presentations, take a case history, examine a patient, carry out special tests and, of course, learn about the running of a real-live business.

One of the benefits of learning in this real-world environment is greater external validity. Given that you are learning in the real world and not in a student clinic within a college or university framework, the training outcomes that you complete are far more likely to be transferable once you become qualified.

A crucial part of your training would include business, accounting, bookkeeping, advertising and marketing, all within the context of an established healthcare clinic. Again, this training would involve both academic work at the affiliate school and observing how this theory is applied in practice together with your mentor.

A structured rotation of mentors could easily be part of the apprenticeship to suit the apprentice's interests, personality, location and experience. Private practice settings don't have to be the only places for hands-on learning; there's much to learn and many sources to learn from. There are hospitals, medical clinics, professional sporting clubs, gyms and continuing professional development courses that could be part of a holistic learning experience. Learning from only one source can stifle the learner; learning from similar and dissimilar professionals and professions creates a much more rounded individual suited to the tasks involved in caring for people.

An apprenticeship may last four years, and apprenticeships are generally competency-based, which means that if you acquire the necessary skills before your training period, you can qualify earlier. All this while being paid to learn.

Once the apprenticeship is completed, many apprentices stay on with their mentors, and others start their own businesses within the field. There are striking similarities between the trades and the allied health industry. We can learn a lot from this well-established and mature process, a model that can efficiently train, support, nurture and invest in the manual therapy profession.

Is it such a long bow to compare a plumber's training with that of a physiotherapist, or a massage therapist's with that of an electrician? The answer is rooted in your epistemology, your worldview, your value systems, and how you see yourself within them. The real issue is not whether you can compare the professions like the trades to those in the allied health field. We can argue about this all day, every day, but that would be missing the point.

What we can, undoubtedly, say though, is that all professions ultimately solve problems for people. So, if we want to solve a problem, the solution doesn't matter to the end user, the patient or the client. All they want is for someone to solve their problem. That someone can be anyone, even someone who has no formal training whatsoever, just a reputation for fixing problems. The fact that we must have training to become manual therapists is a necessity, not for the end-user, but for us.

The customer doesn't care what your undergraduate training involved, whether it was an apprenticeship at a trade school or at an Ivy League university, how many hours you studied or whether you have a diploma or a PhD. It's our egos that get in the way of rational and deliberate thought.

Pie in the sky

DEVELOPING AN ALTERNATIVE to the existing allied health profession training model would demand a massive pivot, one that would certainly twist many an ankle, one that requires rare consensus between schools, universities, regulatory bodies, and the professions and their associations. Given that we don't even accept that there's a problem to solve, how can we expect an alliance of stakeholders first to be formed and subsequently to work together on a solution? The problem can't successfully be tackled alone. That's not to say that the well-meaning and now abundant onboarding training programs offered by larger allied health clinics and centres don't have a place. They certainly do help new grads settle in and support them as they start their careers.

There are quite mature and well-developed postgraduate training schemes out there. Before I sold my clinic in 2014, I had tested and implemented many iterations of a mentoring and support program for the new graduates I employed. The program that worked best had two stages, an undergraduate and a postgraduate stage. We advertised the undergraduate program to the final-year cohorts and invited them to apply for a position with our company.

The system was similar to that used in the legal and accounting professions. We chose undergraduate students who were in their final six months of training and fitted into our business. The deal was that they would come and observe all aspects of our business, not just the treatments, once a week for three months while they were still training. We would then offer the successful newly graduated student a position in the postgraduate mentor program. Once qualified, they could start treating patients. The actual process was very structured. Three afternoons were set aside for the program training, a further three sessions were scheduled where the new graduate would work alone, but I would still be available if required.

I trained two excellent therapists, Tegan and Ed, using our graduate training program, which fast-tracked their real-world private practice experience. After three months, they both enjoyed 80 per cent total patient capacity level. This would have taken any other graduate at least six to twelve months to achieve.

Both new graduates were trained at the same time to maximise the opportunity to learn from each other and make full use of the time available. A training session might start at 2 pm and finish at 6 pm. Receptionists were asked to book my patients every thirty minutes, staggering their booking times every fifteen minutes. Patient A would have an appointment at 2 pm and Patient B would have an appointment at 2:15 pm. All the patients were asked if they would consent to having a colleague attend their appointment for staff training purposes. We used a receptionist script to ensure consistency with what they said. We didn't want any patients to feel uncomfortable. This consent was critical because these patients were paying a premium to see me, not a new graduate. I thought that this step would be our greatest stumbling block because my patients were long-time regulars, who, on paper, would be hard to pass on to the new graduates. Thankfully, I was wrong. The quality of the therapists I had chosen, the fact that they were already known to our patients and staff as undergraduates and my recommendation gave every patient confidence in the system.

So, at 2 pm, I would go in with my patient, confirm that they were still okay for me to bring my new colleague in as part of our training program. I started the treatment, the new grad watched. I introduced the new grad to my patient over the first 15 minutes. At the halfway mark, I would ask if it was okay for the new grad to continue the treatment. If it was, which it was every single time, I would leave the room at 2:15 pm after suggesting what the new grad should be working on and the techniques I would recommend using. I would always confirm with the patient that I would return at the end of the 30-minute treatment to check that they were happy and that we had achieved their treatment goals.

This exact process continued with the second newly qualified graduate at 2:15 pm until I left the second room at 2:30 pm. At 2:30 pm, I would start treating another patient with the first new graduate. This cycle continued for three months, three times a week, until I had passed on almost every one of my patients to the new grads, allowing me to treat fewer patients, as well as support and mentor the new grads. My waiting list freed up, allowing me to bring new patients to the clinic and pass them on to my associates.

As a practice owner, you first need to welcome and accept inevitable change. Think about how you want your working week to look at the end of the mentor program and choose the right people to join your business.

As a new graduate, you need to find the ideal home to perfect your craft, one that will teach you, support you, nurture you and watch you grow into a valued member of a team and the broader profession.

Don't hold on too tight

I MENTIONED TEGAN AND ED in the section 'Pie in the sky'. They were part of my mentorship program in 2010 and were hugely successful in their own rights as osteopaths in my Sports & Spinal Group business and later in their careers. Even though I had heavily invested my time and money in the mentorship program, this didn't and shouldn't mean that as a business owner I have any rights to the product that my program delivers. Holding on too tight is pervasive and entrenched thinking within the mindset of many business owners, and healthcare professionals are not exempt. While I completely understand why a business owner may worry about losing great therapists, it is nevertheless a part of any business. Great people leave but they also join other clinics. Business owners need to think about the bigger picture: you may be losing great talent but someone else, even another industry, will gain from your apprenticeship program and the experience that you've given your trainees.

You need to switch from the negative and unhelpful attitude of loss to one of satisfaction, knowing that you've contributed to that person's professional skills and now they're ready to move on and use their skills elsewhere. Holding on too tight to something you can't control is never helpful for you as the business owner or for the professionals you employ. Let them leave with your blessings. This approach always creates a much better working environment and sets an example for everyone involved in your business.

Tegan Smith now works at one of the largest osteopathic clinics in Melbourne with a great entrepreneur and businesswoman, Jade Harries. I chatted to her in August 2021 about her work and home life. She was about to return to work after maternity leave and was so excited about getting back to work and seeing her patients. Tegan is a lovely person with an engaging personality, and it came as no surprise that she described her patients as her friends. She loves her job, where she gets to help her friends, have fun, and contribute to her community.

You can't help but like Ed from the minute you meet him. He's one of those rare individuals that embodies trust, honesty, and integrity in equal and generous measures. The consistent and incredibly respectful way in which he behaves and communicates with everyone that he meets sets him apart. It is because of these valuable qualities that Ed was highly successful as an osteopath at my clinic and then went on to work at BAT Logic in 2009 as Performance Innovation Director. In 2018 he was appointed Health & Fitness Lead, ANZ & South Asia at Apple. He is a subject matter expert (SME) and evangelist across the Apple pillars of health, fitness and sport for his region.

Here's what Tegan and Ed said about the Osteo Health Group (OHG) Undergraduate Mentorship Program (UGMP) I developed at my practice:

> The biggest benefit of the OHG UGMP is the level of excellence in practice that is expected and continually delivered and the fact that you have a highly experienced and confident mentor who can teach you a lot in a short space of time. I learnt a huge amount during my internship at OHG and I am very grateful. It has made me a much better practitioner and a happy employee as a result. The clinic is very friendly and a dynamic work environment, but its best asset is probably the patient list – this really makes a difference when coming to work.
>
> Dr Tegan Smith, graduate 2009, RMIT University, Bundoora, Victoria, Australia

> I highly recommend the OHG UGMP. This program gave me invaluable experience before I finished uni and it certainly helped me make a confident start to work as a fully qualified Osteopath. The advantage of being in the clinic before starting work is great – you can build your own profile with patients, learn the ins and

outs of the clinic and most importantly get hands-on experience in a real practice. 🙶

Dr Ed Wittich, graduate 2009, AOA Vic Uni Student of the Year
University: Victoria University, Flinders Street Campus, Melbourne,
Victoria, Australia

Before starting the mentorship program, I also employed another great talent, Paul Francis. Paul applied for a job that I advertised with my professional association when he was in Italy, he had moved there to work in clinics in Naples and Rome. We chatted about the job over the phone while Paul was still in Europe. I knew within minutes he was the right fit. I gave him the job at the end of the call.

As soon as he started working at my clinic, he became very popular and quickly built his list. Paul was an incredible outside-the-box thinker. I prepared myself to lose him almost as soon as he arrived. I was delighted to see him achieve his goal of inventing a new piece of equipment designed to help rowers, called a 'foot stretcher' while still working at my clinic. When he showed me an early prototype design, I thought it looked like a smoke alarm, but that demonstrated how little I knew about rowing.

After leaving my clinic in December 2007, Paul started his own business, BAT Logic, in Melbourne. BAT Logic innovates products that allow boats to be customised to rowers and increase performance outcomes.

During the lead up to the London Olympics in 2012, Paul moved to the U.K., where he worked with U.K. Sport in the performance medicine team. Following the Olympics, he joined Nike, becoming one of the global innovation leaders for footwear.

In 2017 he was appointed as the global head of sports science for Adidas. Paul has also consulted to National Football League (U.S.) teams, including the New York Giants, Miami Dolphins and the Atlanta Falcons.

I am so proud of Tegan, Ed, Paul and everyone who has worked in my business. They have achieved so much in their careers so far; I am sure they will continue to contribute as individuals within the organisations they represent and as part of their community.

Learning to fish

CLINICAL PRACTICE, TEACHING AND MENTORING are all equally rewarding. Their settings may be different, but they have one important and critical similarity, which must be appreciated in order to understand the magnitude of their effects.

The familiar quote by Lao-Tzu, the Chinese philosopher, writer and father of Taoism, reads,

> If you give a hungry man a fish, you feed him for a day, but if you teach him how to fish, you feed him for a lifetime.

This is clearly true, but we can take the quote even further. Teaching one person how to perform a manual therapy skill not only provides a lifetime benefit for that person, but the therapist will also benefit their customers, and their customer's families and friends.

The multiplier effects of treating a single patient or teaching a new graduate a skill are profound. By treating a single patient or introducing a new skill to one other healthcare professional, you create exponential ripple effects that are extraordinary. You can potentially help an infinite number of other people, not just the patient you treated or the new grad you teach. The patients you help are part of a wider community, interconnected and dependent upon each other.

Your treatment and your teaching effect are potent: they can influence the health and wellbeing of not just one person, but your patient's entire community network. Each patient's network may include a partner, family member, work colleague, supervisor, teammate or friend. And it gets even better. Each of those human connections has its own separate matrix that multiplies your treatment impact even further.

Head start

IF YOU'RE ABOUT TO GRADUATE or you've recently graduated as a healthcare professional, you have an incredible opportunity to beat the system and win. The best time to start thinking about how you want your business to look is before you're ready to start working in that business or while you still have the time to think and create. While you're in the first few years of your career and even while you're still training, no one expects too much from you, but there's low hanging fruit all around you. Start by imagining that you're already practising rather than waiting for an employer to pluck you from the sea of graduates.

Start by deciding on your business name and structure. A rookie error that many fall prey to is simply to choose a business name that you like the sound of, especially if you add a dot com after that name. The excitement builds quickly as you start to imagine your business name taking on a global importance through branding and identity, while you're holding your phone in one hand and a drink in the other. How easy is that?

All you need now is to find out if anyone has beaten you to this epic business name. No problem, you can find that out in seconds just by typing in the business name into your browser. Lo and behold, you're in luck, no one has that name yet! So, you register your new domain through an online domain registrar.

This ad hoc process is unfortunately all too common because it feels exciting to register your domain name and see it on a web page full of text and photos all about your new business. However, registering your domain name should be one of the last things you should do.

The first thing you should do is talk to an accountant and lawyer about the best business structure for you, now and into the future. Only after you have decided on a business structure should you start thinking about a name. The name is the fun part that you can enjoy after the serious considerations of protection, trademarking, registration, taxation and lodgement is complete. Imagine going through the whole process of creating a website based on a domain name you've registered only to find that the name you're using is also used as a business name?

The best time to be creative and strategic about your career is when you're not thinking about your career or profession. It's challenging to develop ideas when there are other distractions like the part-time job, uni assignments, social gatherings and life's everyday demands. My best ideas have come to me when I'm on holiday or away from work. I'm sure that you've heard the saying that you need to work *on* your business, not *in* your business. Well, that is true, and it's related to what I'm talking about in this section. You need space to allow ideas to flow, clarity to replace chaos, and freedom to overcome limitations and hurdles.

Building a social media presence is a great way to beat the opposition. You can start as early as your final year of training. Why not build your presence on Instagram, Facebook, Twitter and YouTube channels now, before you've seen a single patient? The first objections from the sheep around you will be that you have nothing to say, and no one would want to listen to you if you don't have any professional experience. Nothing could be further from the truth. Everything that you can and want to say when you've already graduated is still valid in the last year of your training.

One of the best ways to start is to develop your story and brand by recording video clips of common exercises, stretches and treatment advice and uploading them to your YouTube channel then link the channel to all the other social media platforms in your business name.

Think about it: almost every patient is given a series of exercises that they promptly forget before they get home after an appointment. How useful would it be for them to have access to a library of exercises that they can watch on any device, at any time? Of course, many off-the-shelf apps can also help your patients without any additional work. However, the big difference is that these sites don't have *you* as the lead actor. There's no link between your brand and the generic apps. If set up correctly, the content library can sit on your site using your colour scheme, fonts, logo and business name. Sending your valued patients off-site is a rookie website error. It's the social equivalent of showing a guest the exit rather than welcoming them through the front door of your home.

Suppose we accept that your website or landing page is your home. A home is where you welcome your guests. Your guests are your customers, who all trust you and rely on your advice and support. Then ask yourself, would I turn a guest away and tell them that I can't help, but I do know someone else who can? No, of course not. You must make those guests, who are your patients, feel welcome whenever they connect with you. Your familiar face, name and voice are vital in retaining the trust of your clients.

Weekly or monthly posts about the thousands of possible topics that your demographic is interested in are easy to create and post. Make the content short and snappy, add music, always include a call to action in every thread, and you have the start of a home worth visiting. Brand any content you create, think about how to make your posts, videos and images different, but above all, make sure they're highly relevant. Use hashtags and handles to help your audience find your content. Add cross-links to all your social media in every communication channel. Every email you send to any other human, patient or not, should include your branded signature, regardless of where they live on the planet.

Relevancy is the most important attribute for all social media content. The best way to determine the relevancy of your posts is to start at the end. The end is the result that you want to achieve. Ask yourself what is the single most important reason for this post? Reasons for posts are not always the same or obvious, there are a variety of possibilities including more likes or followers, more customers, more income or sales, better reviews, higher search engine ranking and positioning yourself as an authority. Depending on your 'why', each post should be curated accordingly, with your end goal in mind.

If, for example your goal, your reason for posting on your social media channels is to become the authority on evidence-based manual treatment approaches for back pain, decide on the metrics that you will use to gauge your degree of success. Arguably this methodology is highly subjective, but you could start with the percentage change in follower numbers over a given period. Obviously, you are assuming that a percentage increase in followers means that your audience is interested in what you have to say. Now tweak your posts, images and hashtags to see how these changes influence your metrics. Record and measure what happens; as the Peter Drucker (1909–2005) saying allegedly goes,

> If you can't measure it, you can't improve it.

My advice is to experiment with all the possible variables that may lead to achieving your intended result and monitor which of these variables have the greatest traction with your audience. Greater traction will ultimately lead to better results.

These simple but effective strategies will allow you to eat from the low hanging fruit before others find the same trees.

My teachers, mentors and resilience

I NOTED EARLIER THAT MY PATIENTS HAVE BEEN MY GREATEST TEACHERS. They have helped me build and grow my manual therapy skills and have widened my knowledge about every conceivable subject you care to mention during our treatment room conversations. I have also been lucky enough to have met some world-class performers who have taught and reminded me about the importance of resilience and constantly raising the bar for myself.

One such person is Dr Jan Dommerholt. Jan is a Dutch-trained physical therapist and the president/CEO of Myopain Seminars, the leading dry needling education provider in the United States. He started teaching dry needling, first in Spain then in the United States in 1997.

I first learnt about Jan in late 2016. He was the first guest on my podcast channel, on which I interviewed experts in dry needling and myofascial pain. In preparation for my podcast, I conducted extensive research to find the key persons of influence within this treatment modality and area of study. You can find all my interviews by searching for **CPD Health Courses Apple Podcasts**.

I found the person I was looking for; Jan was much more than just a key person of influence. His bio is too long to list here, but it can be found on the Myopain Seminars website. One of the many impressive facts about Jan was that he had worked and trained with Dr Janet Travell and Dr David Simons, who authored the seminal book *Myofascial Pain and Dysfunction: The Trigger Point Manual* (1999). The book was an important milestone in our understanding of muscle pain, referral patterns and clinical science. Jan lists some more heavy hitters as his mentors, including Dr Robert Gerwin, Dr Richard S. Materson, Dr Karel Lewit and Dr Peter Baldry.

After I interviewed Jan, I knew that he represented the world standard for dry needling education, and I wanted to learn as much as I could from him. I also wanted to learn and surround myself with the experts that were part of his academic circle. To do that, I would first have to attend all four of his dry needling training courses in the United States and pass the tough final written examination and practical test, to become a Myopain Seminars Certified Myofascial Trigger Point Therapist.

I had launched CPD Health Courses two years earlier. We were growing rapidly and teaching dry needling in every state of Australia, so the timing was right. I knew that to build my dry needling education business, it wasn't good enough just to attend someone else's training course and then call myself a teacher – anyone could do that, and I didn't want to be just anyone – I wanted to learn from the best.

I learnt so much from the whole study and training experience involved with the Myopain Seminars program. Since completing my training, Jan was my guest in Australia when I invited him to present Masterclass Dry Needling training to Australian manual therapists. I have also had the great privilege of teaching alongside him at the 10th World Congress on Myofascial Pain Syndrome and Fibromyalgia Syndrome, held in Bangalore, India, in 2017.

Jan and I have become good friends since our first meeting on air. I will always value his generosity in sharing his knowledge, and I will always respect the standards he has set for himself and others to aspire to.

I have been fortunate in my professional life to have started my osteopathic training at the British School of Osteopathy in London, United Kingdom. I was taught and mentored by some of the greatest manual therapists of that era, who even now command the respect, reverence and recognition of all my peers. I was in the right place at the right time.

I learnt my manual skills from many, including the incredible Professor Laurie Hartman. He, and other faculty members, taught me many things, but above all, they taught me that manual therapy was an art and a craft. Like any craft that I wanted to excel in, I knew that I would have to practise, refine, work and work even harder to reach even an acceptable skill standard. I did this by teaching manual therapy at both Royal Melbourne Institute of Technology University and Victoria University. I found that teaching a skill is one of the most powerful ways to master and refine proficiency and expertise.

The teaching role forces you to learn more than is required of your students; it compels you to examine why you perform every action that's required to accomplish a technique and substantiate everything that you say with evidence in the form of research or demonstration. Great teachers must also inspire their students. My teachers have and continue to inspire me.

You will recall that I have also learnt a great deal from my patients. One person who has always inspired me as well as taught me how incredibly resilient we can be is my good friend and Paralympian, Don Elgin. I first met Don in 1999. The Australian Paralympic Committee had arranged for Paralympians who were preparing for the Sydney Olympics to receive osteopathic care from any osteopath wanting to participate in the program. Don lived nearby and called to make his first appointment. I knew we would be lifetime friends from the minute I met him. Over the first few treatments he explained his story. One anecdote he shared with me has stayed in my mind ever since.

Don was first introduced to the idea of competing at the Paralympics by his best friend at school, Craig Kelly, when he was fourteen years old. Craig asked Don an important question as they sat at the back of the classroom one day. As it happens, this question was a pivotal moment in Don's thinking.

Craig asked Don if he'd thought about entering the Paralympics. In Craig's words, "They're just like the Olympics but for disabled people." Don's response was classic, "Yeah, but there's one problem – I'm not disabled."

Prior to this question, Don had never considered himself disabled, all he knew was that there was an issue with his leg, but he had an artificial one, which meant he could do almost anything as well as the other guys, sometimes even better. "No big deal."

That ten-year-old boy who was born with one and a half legs and whose fingers were stuck together went on to represent Australia and compete at four World Championships (1994, 1998, 2002 and 2006), a Commonwealth Games (2014) and three Paralympic Games (1996, 2000 and 2004).

Don is married to Denise, his first wife as he likes to refer to her at every opportunity. I have been to their home, met their children, their parents, brothers, sisters and friends, many times. The Elgin family and everyone connected with them are one of the most loving, supportive and generous families I know. They continually demonstrate the importance of family through their daily actions; they don't just talk about what they would do if someone asked for help; they do it. They are the sort of family that would welcome a complete stranger to their home, offer a kind word, something to eat and a place to sleep. No questions asked. They are strong, resilient, kind and always humble.

An example of Don's humility was when he returned from the 2004, Athens Paralympic Games having won Silver in the Men's 4 × 400 m T42–46 relay event. At the first opportunity to thank me for looking after him in preparation for the games, Don arrived at my clinic with a gift. It wasn't the traditional bottle of wine or a box of chocolates. Don presented me with his Paralympic Silver medal. That's all I need to say for you to know who Don and the Elgin family are and what they mean to me.

Jacqui Cooper is another person that I would list as one of my friends and someone who has shaped my thinking and behaviours. Don referred her to me as a patient. As it happened, she lived near my clinic and was in need of treatment as she prepared to represent Australia in Aerial Skiing at the Vancouver, Canada Winter Olympics in 2010. I've met thousands of people, but no one with the single-minded, focused mental toughness that she has. Jacqui has used her strong mental character to become a World Champion athlete despite countless injuries as a result of her training and competing at the highest level.

Jacqui has competed in 139 World Cup Events, nine World Championships and been selected on five Winter Olympic Teams. Jacqui competed in Vancouver in February 2010 and, as such, became the first Australian woman in history (summer or winter Olympics) to represent Australia at five Games. Her record five world titles, 39 World Cup medals, 24 World Cup wins, and three major World Championship medals has left Jacqui as the greatest aerial skier of all time (man or woman), an achievement that will remain unbeaten for decades.

My knowledge about running a business has grown through practice, hours of reading, attending courses and joining online marketing and advertising training. I've spent a lot of time and money learning from the best teachers that I could find, some of them I've engaged as my mentors to help me with small and large projects over the past thirty-five years.

I have observed one common thread between all my mentors and teachers: their process of continual grind and relentless practice, trying to improve by even the smallest of margins, every day. Just like a saving mindset, every bit counts. The smallest daily margins of improvement all add up and compound into a wealth of mental strength and life experience. Over time, problems that were previously challenging become imperceptible blips on the radar, hardly worthy of mention.

I have found that the best way to learn is to fail and fail frequently. By failing, I learn. The more I fail, the more I learn. I love the challenge of solving problems when things don't go the way I would like or expect them to go. The experience of overcoming challenges, small or large, is like forging steel; it hardens you, making you more resilient and able to meet the next challenge better prepared and more experienced.

One person who has researched the power of failure and how it can help us become more resilient is a number one *New York Times* best-selling author and psychologist, Angela Duckworth. I have read her book, *Grit: The Power of Passion and Perseverance* three times, because I have learnt something new every time I have read it.

Everyone copes well when things are going well in their life, but the true measure of a person's character is how well they cope with life when it is not going their way. In her book, Angela describes how highly successful people behave. She interviewed hundreds of leaders in business, the arts, athletics, journalism, academia, medicine and law. She asked them:

> Who are the people at the top of your field?
> What makes them special and what are they like?

There were many common characteristics that came from the study, some were industry specific, and many could be applied generally.

Some of the commonalities include the ability to stick it out when you're met with failure and not fall apart. A really interesting insight was that high achievers were satisfied with being unsatisfied. For these leaders, the chase was as satisfying as the capture. Summing up the qualities of a high achiever, Angela explains that these exemplars are highly resilient and hardworking, they knew what they wanted, had not only direction but determination. The combination of passion and perseverance made these high achievers special. They had grit. If you want to know where you are on the grit scale, you can take Angela's grit questionnaire, which is available on her website: **angeladuckworth.com**.

Like any business, the healthcare business is all about solving problems, day in and day out. Anyone could run a business if everything went to plan, but as we know, nothing always goes to plan, not in business or any other part of our lives.

By solving problems, overcoming challenges and making hundreds of mistakes, I have learnt many important lessons; the take-home message is that success is about how well you deal with failure.

'Plane' sailing – not

MY CESSNA-150 LINED UP behind the Monarch Airlines Boeing 720 on runway 26 at Luton Airport in Bedfordshire, UK. The international departure in front of me was headed for one of the many charter flight destinations in Europe that afternoon and I was off to the training area where I would practise medium-level turns from straight and level flight.

For as long as I can remember, I wanted to learn to fly an aeroplane. As I sat in the left-hand seat, the position assigned to the captain of a flight, I imagined that I had swapped places with the captain of the plane ahead of us, which was about to take off.

My instructor, who sat next to me, was really in charge, had his head down while signing off the maintenance release and clearing us for the short flight ahead. I wasn't sure if he was deliberately ignoring me in an attempt to calm my nerves or he really hadn't noticed that I was seconds away from take-off into controlled airspace, for what was only my third flying lesson.

At age 17, I completed only a handful of one-hour flying lessons while still living in the United Kingdom. I looked forward to every lesson, counting the days until I could afford another. Unfortunately, financial reality caught up with me – I could no longer afford the lessons. I had a part-time job washing pots and pans in a local restaurant and even together with my savings from the summer before, it wasn't enough. The year was 1980 and it took me about four weeks to save enough money for a one-hour flying lesson, not including travel costs to and from the airport. I vowed that one day, when I had a real job, I would complete my training.

My opportunity to resume my flight training presented itself when I emigrated to Australia with my wife in 1987. Flying lessons were so much cheaper than in the UK, but so was almost everything else. Don't get me wrong, it wasn't that cheap that it was comparable to a round of golf or hiring a tennis court for an hour. Given that my wife and I had great jobs as osteopaths and we had no children, flying was certainly a luxury but one that was affordable at that time in our lives. It was time to try and achieve my childhood dream again.

It was never my intention to switch careers and become a commercial pilot, at least not at the beginning of my flying journey. I have always been open to any possibility at any time – you just never know what can happen and where new doors might lead you. I wasn't scared of having a go and seeing what happens next; after all I had already gambled by leaving the place where I grew up, went to school, made many friends and of course where my family lived.

My never say never attitude probably comes from my mother. If I said, "Mum, I want to be an astronaut on the space shuttle", she would probably reply with, "You can be anything you want to be, why don't you apply?"

I met a wonderful flying instructor, Martin Waite out at Coldstream Airport in Melbourne's Yarra Ranges. It was convenient for me as I had a job as an associate at a nearby clinic in Forest Hill. Martin is the calmest man I have ever met, and I attribute almost all of my flying achievements to his amazing ability to make the complex, simple. I loved his common-sense approach to almost any challenge.

They say that no one ever forgets the day they go solo. I am no exception. It was a wet winter's afternoon, and I was doing circuits in the Cessna-152, landing on the slippery, muddy grass strip we called a runway. Circuits are a flight training exercise that involves taking off, a climbing turn, levelling off, flying parallel to the runway, a descending turn, lining up with the runway and finally, landing. The landing is called a 'touch and go' because as soon as you land you must repeat the whole exercise again by retracting the flaps, adding the power then taking off again. This co-ordinated and ordered process is repeated until all the elements are achieved safely and accurately to the satisfaction of your flying instructor.

Every student pilot knows when their instructor thinks they are ready to go solo, because immediately before they attempt a solo circuit, their instructor will say the following sentence on the penultimate final approach: "Make this one a full-stop." It's at that time that you realise that your instructor thinks it's time, time for you to go solo, just you in the plane, armed with your newly acquired skills and confidence.

While I performed my first solo circuit, I did not think for one second about the consequences of getting it wrong, Martin had trained me well. By achieving this lifetime ambition, I had gone from unconscious incompetence to unconscious competence. I completed the single circuit, parked the aircraft and walked into the clubrooms to be met by Martin and the school's Chief Flying Instructor who threw a tea towel at me, and said, "Take that, you'll need it to wipe the smile off your face." We all laughed together, knowing that like many before me, something special had happened that afternoon. Even though I only had a handful of hours recorded in my logbook, I now belonged to a special group. It didn't matter how much experience I had, I was now a pilot, I was one of them and I was hooked. My apprenticeship had just begun.

Hooked is a little bit of an understatement. Over the next few years, I completed my initial training, which involved flying training, written examinations, flight tests and endorsements. Once I gained a Private Pilot's Licence I just kept going. By 1996, I had a Commercial Pilot's Licence and passed the written Airline Transport Pilot's Licence examinations, which covered flight planning, loading and performance, navigation, meteorology, aerodynamics, and systems and air law based on a Boeing-727 aircraft. I couldn't stop, I was addicted.

I realised that if I became a flight instructor, I could not only fly more but I would even get paid to fly. It couldn't get any better. Well, what was I going to do? Of course, I started training to become a Flight Instructor at Moorabbin airport and not long after I became a newly qualified Grade 3 instructor.

I was lucky because the school I did my training at was awarded a contract to teach Indonesian students to fly, taking them from school leavers to commercial pilots over a twelve-month period.

Even though by that time I was starting my own practice from home, I loved the challenge of teaching flying in the morning and treating patients the afternoon. I remember buying one of the first mobile phones on the market, fondly referred to as the Motorola brick due its weight and hefty size. I needed a phone because I had to keep my clinic going and take appointments, sometimes on a cross-country flight training exercise.

I met so many wonderful students who all shared my passion for flying. I made a flip chart of my lesson plans, constantly tweaked my teaching methods and practised presentations in front of my family and friends. The role of flight instructor taught me a lot about teaching to a variety of students, all with different educational backgrounds and experiences.

Unlike the formal teaching setting that I had been used to at a university, it wasn't a level playing field. I taught business owners, plumbers, carpenters, electricians, young people straight from school, a hairdresser, an architect and even a seventy-three-year-old grandfather who just wanted to go solo, nothing else. As a flight instructor it was now my turn to say those immortal words to my students, jump out of the cockpit and watch as they would taxi off to their solo flight.

It wasn't long before I became a Grade 1 instructor, the highest level of flight instructor, which gave me greater responsibilities in line with my flying experience. It was after I had achieved the jewel in the crown for all pilots, a multi-engine command instrument rating that I realised I must set a new goal for myself to make the most out of my investment in my training, study and accumulated flight hours. The multi-engine command instrument rating enables pilots to fly using only the instruments in the cockpit without reference to the horizon or land features. The skills that are part of this training allow a pilot to fly in cloud or when weather reduces visibility below the required minimums.

There was a lot to consider: I had a fast-growing home practice, my wife Louise and I now had a two-year-old daughter, beautiful Grace. No longer were we fancy free and able to do what we wanted, when we wanted.

Louise has always been my greatest supporter – she knows that when I put my mind to something, nothing can stop me. I wanted to see where my flying would lead me and how far I could go, I knew I would always have my osteopathic skills, but I may never have the opportunity to explore a career in aviation again, once we had more children and a busy practice. It was a chance of a lifetime.

At the time, the best place for me to get more experience as a pilot and land a job with an airline was Darwin, 3741 kilometres away in the Northern Territory. Within weeks, we had packed up our bags and leased our home out for twelve months. I resigned from my flying instructor job at Civil Flying School, Moorabbin, and we were on our way up north.

I will never forget the first morning waking up on the floor of a friend's Darwin apartment, as Louise and I listened to the strange new bird song and the sounds of insects, feeling the intense humidity and heaviness of the tropical air. We were thinking the same thing: OMG, what have we done? I found out, very soon.

The Darwin experience was one of the most challenging of my life, but I am still so glad that I chose to risk it all to see what I could achieve. My first task was to find a job, any job. I knew that finding a flying job wasn't going to be easy; every pilot from down south who had aspired to fly for an airline one day was in Darwin competing against the next person for their first big break.

Darwin Airport's charter operators all knew that pilots from the southern states came to the Northern Territory for one thing and one thing only: a flying job of any description so that they could accumulate hours as a commercial pilot, then leave when they get a job with one of the big boy airlines in anywhere but Darwin. Everyone in the aviation industry knew the deal, the operators needed the pilots, and the pilots needed the experience. It was a symbiotic relationship that was begrudgingly tolerated.

Pilots would arrive at eight in the morning, armed with a resume and their logbook. The daily routine began by knocking on every hangar door or operator's office. It would have been easier to get an appointment to speak with Elvis. Some would be polite and suggest somewhere else you could try, and others would simply brush you off with the silent treatment. I learnt a lot about handling rejection in my first month.

I was lucky, I was offered a job shortly after arriving, it turned out to be the only job I was offered in the eight months we spent in Darwin. It wasn't a flying job, but it was at the airport. I was a gofer. Yes, that's right, go for this, go for that. Rob was my boss, he was the chief engineer at what was one of the largest helicopter operators on the aerodrome, Lloyd Helicopters. Lloyd had a contract with the oil and gas companies to fly workers out to the rigs in the Timor Sea.

At first, I enjoyed the job and the greater levels of responsibility I was given. I had to work to earn money, but I used every bit of spare time to knock on the same doors and wait for one to open and get my first charter flight. In the meantime, I swept the hangar floor, washed helicopters, ran errands, picked up supplies from hardware stores, filed documents, taxied staff around the airport and, one day, I actually got to take a trip in the impressive AS 332 Super Puma helicopter.

After a few months of constant networking, attending functions where I was told someone who knew someone might be there, and the daily grind of knocking on operator's doors I realised I had a problem. I was too old and had too much flying experience, I was the wrong fit. I looked around and could see that the only pilots getting the charter jobs were ones in their early twenties without any family, with two hundred to three hundred hours. They were mobile, which was very handy for an operator, who could station you in an Aboriginal community like Maningrida for twelve months and you would be eternally grateful for the opportunity to fly every day, racking up valuable flying experience.

Time was running out, my job at Lloyd Helicopters was coming to an end and we were about to run out of money. I had to make a decision: find another job and stay or return to Melbourne empty handed.

I decided on the latter. I had given it a good go. I wasn't going to get any younger and my 1250 hours of flying experience wasn't going to change. I couldn't put my wife and daughter through even more stress and uncertainty. We left Darwin and returned to Melbourne eight months after we had arrived.

Small problem – we couldn't get back into our house because our tenants were there for another four months. So, we had nowhere to live and I had no job, therefore no income. Fortunately, friends of ours offered us a bedroom to live in until we could get back on our feet. Deidre and Brian McDonough not only offered us a roof over our heads but a valuable job. They had a family business installing insulation batts into roofs. For the next few months, I would wake up with all the tradesmen in Melbourne at six am, jump into the van with Brian, tow the trailer to their factory, load the required number and specification of pink batts into the trailer then drive to our first job. Armed with a long stick, a head torch and knee pads, Brian would lean a ladder against the gutter, climb up to the roof line, lift just enough tiles for me and the bags of insulation batts to squeeze into the roof space. Once that job was complete, I had to lay the batts in to every corner of the roof while avoiding stepping onto the plasterboard ceiling. Brian would then go to another job and come back when I was finished. I was grateful for the work, don't get me wrong, but it was physically strenuous and mentally tiring.

Dealing with the mental challenge was the greatest lesson I've ever learnt. Here I was, an osteopath after four years of study, I had earned the respect of my patients and peers, people used to pay me for my professional advice and treatment, I had taught undergraduates at one of Australia's finest universities, and now look at me. My ego had taken a good battering, I had to deal with feelings of disappointment, shame, embarrassment, but most of all I had to accept that I had failed. There was no dressing this up into something else to make it more palatable; I had failed myself and my family. That's how I felt – this was a painful lesson.

As often happens with me, when I'm least expecting it, an idea pops into my head, gets the feasibility check over and then pops out for wider approval shortly after. This one day came months after becoming, even if I say so myself, quite a bit quicker at laying insulation even in the most difficult of spaces. I remember doing a job in a suburb close to where our home was, I was about to drive into a petrol station that I used to go to all the time. I caught a glimpse of a patient that I used to treat just as I entered the station, my immediate and involuntary gut instinct was to continue driving past the bowsers as quickly as possible for fear of the patient seeing me in my insulation speckled tracksuit bottoms, runners and baseball cap. I kept on driving and filled up somewhere else.

It was now almost Christmas and our parents, knowing of our fate wanted us to come back to the United Kingdom to spend the festive period and New Year with them. We had no money for three air fares, but I couldn't tell my parents that. What if I applied for a credit card on the basis of owning, well, having a mortgage, on a Bayside home? I could then pay for the tickets using the available credit on the card once we got to the UK. We could stay with family until the end of January when we could return to our home and I could start up my practice? Louise approved the plan and we packed our bags for the UK within a couple of weeks of making the decision.

The trip took on special significance, not only because of the support of our families but the time I now had to reflect on what went wrong with the Darwin plan and, more importantly what I had to do to fix it.

I had learnt so much about myself over the preceding twelve months. Failure had borne greater resilience. The lessons I learnt will stay with me for the rest of my life. One analogy I use to explain the Darwin experience is that the journey had pushed my body and my mind to new limits of tolerance. Like any training that takes us to new boundaries, my new range was much wider, I was able to take bigger hits and still recover, sink to deeper depths and still bob up breathing, but most of all the experience had provided valuable perspective on what a real challenge was. From then on, any problem I encountered was nothing like the Darwin experience, it was well within my range of tolerance.

Everyday business problems became minor interruptions and of little significance, barely raising a blip on the radar. The lessons that I had learnt were amplified further because the consequences of my decisions and actions didn't just affect me; they affected my family, the collateral effect on the most important people in my life meant that the lessons were etched deeper into my memory and will never be forgotten.

The financial cost of the flying journey was well into six figures, if you include the inevitable loss of income as well as the cost of training. Having said that, learning to fly, moving to Darwin and putting my osteopathy career on hold wasn't a waste of time. I still have no regrets; the money and time was well spent, and I have many friends who did become commercial pilots and are now employed by an airline. I'm so proud of their achievements, I know how hard they've worked and the sacrifices they've made.

The aviation industry and becoming a commercial pilot has taught me many things apart from the teaching skills I mentioned earlier, I also learnt about the importance of safety, apprenticeship, partnership, systems, processes, teamwork and trust. I have used these lessons every day in my business and osteopathy practice.

Thinking on paper

JOURNALING IS ONE OF THE ESSENTIAL HABITS that you must schedule each day or every week. One way to describe the benefits of journaling is to liken it to a mental sieve. I pour my thoughts about the events, interactions and outcomes of my day or week into the empty sieve. The thoughts sit and mix on one side of the perforated barrier, and I wonder whether they'll make it into print as part of my journal. The gems of thought condense on the other side of the barrier as single words or a sentence.

According to a paper by Baikie and Wilhelm, 'Emotional and physical health benefits of expressive writing' (2005), there are many health benefits to reflective practice, including fewer stress-related visits to the doctor, improved immune-system functioning, reduced blood pressure, improved lung function, improved liver function, fewer days in hospital, improved mood/effect, feeling of greater psychological wellbeing, and reduced depressive symptoms before examinations.

A less scientific reference, but one that is still worthy of note, is a wonderful book that I highly recommend, *Tools of Titans* by Tim Ferriss (2016). The book is a record of daily habits and advice from world-class performers in every possible field of study, sporting endeavour and business. Almost everyone included in the book journals daily or regularly and recommends its use for its positive mental benefits.

My journal has evolved over the years and now takes the form of focused thought that I record under constant headings to serve as a prompt later. I have three headings; each is designed to guide my thought process and focus for that day or longer.

Simultaneously writing or typing and thinking or reading helps me record and reflect on my daily experiences. My preference is to keep a digital journal rather than use pen and paper because I can search for dates, names and keywords quickly and easily. I've found that allocating five to ten minutes for journaling every day is right for me. I don't write down everything that comes into my head, just what feels essential, significant, surprising, engaging or thought-provoking.

I don't always journal every day, but I always reserve time for thought. My thinking time is usually at the gym, in the car, or doing something that requires no extra mental exertion.

My journal headings have changed over the years to suit my circumstances, new business ventures, priorities and the areas of my life that I wanted to work on the most. Currently, my three headings are 'Word', 'Quote', 'Action'.

The prompt that sits under the heading 'Word' might be a new word that I came across, either while reading my social media feed, a research article or news report or listening to a book; or it might even be someone's name. I may want to memorise it, learn its meaning, or I just like the word. Sometimes, the term is from a language other than English. If it isn't English, it will probably be of Greek, Latin or French origin. I love etymology, especially from the root languages. Next to the word may be its definition or how it might be used in a sentence, or its relevance to me at that time. Right now, my word is 'solipsism'. Why solipsism? I came across the word in the book *God Is Not Great* by Christopher Hitchens (2017). The word struck me when I heard it in the audiobook version because of its intensity.

Under the heading 'Quote' I write a sentence or statement that got me thinking and strikes me as worthy of further scrutiny and critical examination. My current selection is from Greg McKeown's second book, *Effortless* (2021). Greg poses the question,

> What would this look like if it were easy?

Greg would probably admit that he's not the first person to posit this thought-provoking but straightforward question. Anything that I include under the heading 'Quote' will have interrupted my thoughts on any given day and caused me to reflect further.

My final heading is 'Action'. The prompt under the heading 'Action' may be something that I have set as a goal, a relationship I've neglected and would like to re-establish or a task that I must prioritise on that day, week or month.

The prompts under the headings, 'Word', 'Quote' and 'Action' are just the starting points for further thought that day or days, but more often than not, I've realised that I receive the greatest return when I discuss my words and quotes with others. I choose my moments, but it never fails to surprise me how others can have an entirely different angle on what I mistakenly thought was a reasonably concrete insight. It's exciting to witness and incredibly refreshing to accept that I may have missed the point entirely.

In addition to digital journaling, I also use my phone to set a reminder about any or all of my prompts. Currently, I have a daily reminder that appears at 9 am every day and has popped up on my phone and laptop screen for the past year. It simply reads, 'Be curious'. I am still learning this vital lesson. Journaling has helped me challenge my naturally assumptive mind and continue my probable lifetime struggle and attempt to remain curious about everything.

Like many of the suggestions in this book, I recommend that you start while you're still training, although it's never too late; the earlier, the better. Even if you're at the start of your undergraduate course, studying many of the drier rather than the more relevant clinical subjects, you'll still benefit from a daily journal entry.

Capturing your thoughts, feelings, achievements, learnings, problems, successes and failures is a wonderful way of seeing the recurring patterns that shape your life. By keeping a journal, we are forced to think. Thinking is the precursor to change; change is the start of opportunity and infinite possibility.

You're in sales

WHETHER YOU WORK FOR SOMEONE as an associate, partner or contractor, whether you have your own clinic or health centre, you're in business. The business of human interactions is a sales business. You're a salesperson first and a therapist second. The quicker you adjust your mindset to that order, the better. You see, most therapists believe the opposite is true. Nothing could be further from the truth. You need to be able to sell *you* and *your* 'product' first while standing out in an increasingly crowded, hostile, changing and often unforgiving market.

You need to think of your product as a new idea or invention that you created. Even if your creation was the best thing since the advent of the bicycle, unless you can sell that idea, it's dead in the water and will stay there with all the other unrealised ideas and inventions.

The trouble is that sales have been associated with arguably some of the ugliest words in the dictionary, such as 'money', 'cash', 'deals', 'free', 'discounts' and 'bargains'. Healthcare professionals are way above that, aren't they? That mindset is old-fashioned nonsense and certainly a fallacy.

Surgeons, barristers, engineers, teachers, nurses and dentists are among the most highly rated professions by the public; yet they are all in sales. Each of the people within these professions is selling something. They sell an opinion, advice, an idea, an analysis, a plan, a thought or an option. We, the customers, have to decide if we want to buy. We base our decision to buy on the quality of the sales proposition. Buying and selling rarely involve the exchange of money.

Sales don't just happen when you go shopping; sales occur every time someone solves a problem for a customer. In your case, the customer is your patient or client. Their problem is that they can't work, play golf, or pick their baby up. You make a sale every time you provide a plan, give advice, provide a treatment or try to relieve their pain. The patient pays you because you have attempted to solve their problem.

Selling feelings

WE, AS HEALTHCARE PROFESSIONALS, are in the business of selling feelings. To think that patients come to see you because they want you to correct their posture, crack their neck, dry needle their traps, massage their muscles, give them a handout with the reps and sets for a particular exercise plan, or give them advice about how they should cope with their chronic pain condition is wrong. You're missing the point, and you're underselling yourself.

None of these technical or manual skills are decisive factors that patients consider when they shop around. They buy how your technical, academic and manual skills make them feel. They are receptive to everything you have to offer before they even enter your practice or clinic. They begin their engagement as soon as they start thinking about their next appointment, which could be when they confirm their appointment or call your rooms to make an appointment. It could even begin with someone else reminding them that they have a treatment booked with you tomorrow.

I am the Director of CPD Health Courses, a dry needling education provider for healthcare professionals. We currently present more dry needling courses than any other company in Australia, and before the COVID-19 pandemic, we were also teaching our courses in the United Kingdom.

At every dry needling course that we present, we always say that if you can't sell these techniques to your patients, then you're wasting your time on the course. You might as well leave right now. We'll remind every therapist that comes to our courses that they are salespeople first and therapists second. They need to understand this fundamental, undeniable fact.

You might be thinking that by 'selling', I mean that you're selling your skills as a therapist. You're selling an amazing technique you've learnt, advice about a unique exercise program to strengthen the lower back or perhaps your time and knowledge about how to manage a chronic condition. These certainly are valuable and practical skills to impart, but that's not what you're selling, and it certainly isn't what your patients want. Patients want and deserve the emotions and feelings that delivering these skills generate.

Have you ever stayed up long enough to watch a few minutes on a TV shopping channel? It's certainly worth the effort if you want to learn how they sell hundreds of items that you can easily buy at any shop or online website. The standard set-up is that you have two people talking about each item, carefully chosen to mirror the ideal buyer's exact demographic. TV shopping channels sell many things, including clothing, kitchen appliances, jewellery, white goods and, of course, home gym equipment.

Each product's function is irrelevant. All knives cut tomatoes, all fridges cool your drinks, and all gym weights are either light, medium or heavy. The brightly coloured, breathable cotton dress you can buy right now for three easy payments of only $19.99 plus free shipping will 'give you the feeling that you're on holiday every time you wear it'. Every day is a holiday. The latest Ab gym workout machine, 'backed by science and the latest research', is guaranteed to give you a rippling six-pack in just twelve weeks. Why is this appealing? It's not because you love doing endless crunches and going on a low carb diet. It's because you'll love the feeling of pride as onlookers admire your tight and athletic body at the beach this summer.

Whether we're talking about the fridge, jewellery, clothing, Ab machine or indeed a neck treatment, none are related directly to the product itself but to the evocation of a feeling that is promised once you make that purchase. Once you start to abandon the belief system that falsely positions your academic and technical skills above those of the emotions and feelings your customer is searching for, logic prevails in all your future decision-making processes. Business becomes easier when you know the objective. A clear signal prevails over the noise of confusion. Finally, you realise that your true purpose is to sell feelings using the technical skills and knowledge you learnt during your training.

All ears

IT'S YOUR SECOND WEEK IN PRACTICE. You've arrived at the clinic, greeted the receptionist on duty that morning, turned the computer on in your treatment room then logged in to the patient management system. As you browse through the day's list of patients, you see an entry at the start of the list, "URGENT – Ms Joan Parker – Worse after treatment, see reception staff."

That's the dreaded message that causes a sickening feeling over the solar plexus of every healthcare practitioner. It doesn't matter how long you've been in practice, that's the message no one likes to receive. When it happens, you hope that it never happens again, but it will.

As the knot tightens in the pit of your stomach, you walk out to get the message from the receptionist. You feel as if she's judging you and her respect and confidence in you has dropped in the space of two days. She knows that you've got one of those messages. No words are spoken, but both you and the receptionist know why you're at the front desk. A fleeting but disturbing thought enters your mind. The receptionist, who is also the gatekeeper at your workplace, will never trust you with another new patient again. Your list will dry up, and you'll have to get a new job somewhere very far away. Far away from Ms Parker and the gatekeeper. All these thoughts within minutes of reading a few words.

So, she gives you the message. Of course, she knows what's written on that piece of paper. It's been sitting there since your last shift, two days earlier for every subsequent receptionist to read. As if that wasn't embarrassing enough, all the practitioners on that day have also seen the 'urgent' message for you on your patient list through the convenience of modern-day patient record-keeping software.

You call Ms Parker, who tells you that she's never felt worse after treatment in all her years of coming to the clinic. She ends the conversation by booking in to see your boss, who normally treats her. How do you feel? Shell-shocked and gutted like many who've come before you and have experienced this unfortunate event. It can happen to any of us, experienced as well as inexperienced practitioners.

This infrequent event is an excellent opportunity to test your communication skills, your ability to listen, your choice of effective vocabulary, and your understanding of treatment room choreography. More about choreography later. This is one of those fail moments you want to welcome every time it happens. Fortunately, I've had a few of these experiences, given that I've probably given about 80,000 treatments in my career to date. The first one of these wasn't one that I relished, I must say. I still remember thinking that this might be the end of my short-lived career. As it turned out, I still see the same patient now, and they've referred many others since. That's the other thing – situations and adverse events are never as bad as we make them out to be at the time.

What I learnt from this first adverse treatment event is a crucial lesson about listening. I realised that my talk to listen to ratio changed from 90:10 to 10:90 in these situations. Talk 10 per cent and listen 90 per cent. A 2011 *Harvard Business Review* article titled 'How to listen' by Peter Bregman suggests that we should listen ten times more than we talk, 10:1, especially with customers.

The last time I remember having to deal with a patient who felt worse after treatment was a few years ago now, but I still remember it as if it was yesterday. I remember it because when the patient walked into my room, I knew I would be okay. I knew the outcome would be what we both wanted. I provided the patient with the answers they wanted and the pain relief they were looking for, without blame, without taking it personally, and really caring about how they felt. All I did was listen more than I spoke.

One of the greatest lessons you can learn and learn fast is that we're all the same. In the context of a patient who hasn't responded as expected, they're usually in fear. There's always a reason for the fear, which for us as the expert may appear irrational, but we would act in a similar way if we were in their shoes. Learn to stand in their shoes and ask yourself what you would do.

Finding gold

ONE OF THE ESSENTIAL ATTRIBUTES of any practitioner is a great attitude. That's not to say that being technically gifted is not important. Both ability and attitude are important. However, attitude is more valuable than ability. After all, there's no point in having bucketloads of ability but a lousy attitude.

In the seminal book, *Good to Great* (2009) by the iconic American business author, Jim Collins, there's a simple but beautiful quote:

> Good is the enemy of great.

Just six words but they force you to think for hours about their meaning to you and your business processes.

What Collins means is that you could just go about your business as everyone else does, accept that some patients may not come back, accept that you may not have a complete list every day, accept that you will never have a waiting list of people wanting to see you, accept that your reputation as a practitioner may never be greater than the other practitioners in your area. You could just accept that good is good enough. However, if great rather than good is your goal, you're heading for a world-class performance in your career.

By choosing to invest in your knowledge and skills, you've made a choice, the choice that good is not good enough. Great is your destiny. Good is your enemy. Too many people opt for good when great is so much more rewarding for you and your patients.

Let's think about an experience we are all familiar with: the new patient consultation. Although the new patient consultation is being used in this example, all the information and advice can be and should also be applied to a repeat treatment or a re-examination. The procedures are exactly the same, and they have the same degree of importance, although a new patient consultation does carry special significance.

New patients are precious, precious multiplier opportunities that carry enormous potential benefits to you and your practice if you invest in them and look after them. One slip-up, and you could lose not only that patient but many potential referrals from them as well.

In the following sections, I will cover everything you need to know about a new patient consultation, from the first contact in the waiting room to the closure script at the end of their treatment. Each component of a new patient consultation is a small step towards the final goal: the creation of a lifelong customer who can't wait to tell their family and friends about their experience, your treatment and how much better they feel.

The new patient consultation is the foundation for an infinite number of future consultations by that patient and others they will refer to you. In business terms, your new patient is known as a 'lead'. The marketing pathway starts with a lead which becomes a 'prospect', then finally a 'customer'. A lead is someone who responds to your advert or perhaps your signage.

At the lead stage, there is only one-way communication from you to them. Once you contact the lead, two-way communication is initiated, which is when they become a prospect. A prospect is someone who has the potential to become a customer. A customer is created once they buy from you.

The lead is interested in your product, but they haven't bought it yet; they've made the appointment, but they haven't paid yet. If this was an online shopping experience, the lead has arrived at your website because of your advertising, they're browsing your products, but they haven't added any to their cart or checked out. Similarly, the lead has arrived at your practice because of a referral or your online presence.

When the lead makes their first move and contacts your business, you have an opportunity to convert them from a lead into a prospect and finally into a lifelong patient or customer. Lifelong patients are your best and most valuable customers because they will tell everyone about you and your business.

Seth Godin, the American author of *Unleashing the Ideavirus* (2000), calls these people 'sneezers'. Sneezers are the patients who tell their family, friends and work colleagues about you, and everyone believes them. They spread your idea among their community network, which can be far and wide. The best part about their infection is that it's free. According to Godin, there are two types of sneezers, 'promiscuous' and 'powerful'.

A promiscuous sneezer sells your idea for personal gain; there has to be something in it for them. The gain can be money, discounts, favours or other inducements. An example might be when a patient attends your clinic for treatment – they like what you do and how you do it. You fix them, and they get back to playing football in record time – an excellent result for you and them. They like your idea, the idea being the way you do things in your clinic. You seize upon this opportunity and offer them a free or discounted treatment in return for each new patient they refer to your clinic over the next twelve months. The return for the promiscuous sneezer doesn't have to be cash; it may just be something like preferential appointment times or discounted appointment fees.

Powerful sneezers, on the other hand, cannot be bought; they sneeze by setting trends. In our world of healthcare, these people are the ones who already have a degree of authority in their community, and others look for their lead. Once they experience your treatment, they sneeze and spread the idea based on their pre-existing level of power and influence. They're the shepherds, not the flock.

You can identify both types of sneezers by carefully listening to what they say to you, your reception staff, your colleagues and in the case of powerful sneezers, following them on their social media profiles. The two patients that I discussed in the section 'Differentiators' are great examples of promiscuous sneezers.

Powerful sneezers are hard to come by, but highly valuable to your business. They include medical doctors and specialists, local politicians, elite athletes and community leaders.

You must work hard if you want to earn the trust and reap the rewards from either type of sneezer. You will quickly work out who these people are by collecting the data about the referral source of your new patients. Once identified, sneezers must be nurtured, all the time understanding what they feed on, personal gain or growing authority.

It doesn't matter which type of sneezer you attract. As long as it's organic and unforced, the effect on your business will be remarkable. All you have to do is to make sure that your idea is worth spreading.

I have analysed the sneezers and the people they sneezed upon at my practice between 2001 and 2011. For these ten years, I looked at specific metrics, including the number of times they attended my clinic, the number of other patients they referred, the total number of visits, and the average spend over the ten years. Based on my average fees during this period, the value of one sneezer was around $10,625. That's just one sneezer. I calculated that forty-three patients had referred twenty-five other people or more in the ten years I studied. I was staggered to realise the value of this organic exponential growth. It was priceless.

Now, factor in that most therapists are in practice for thirty or forty years. I certainly don't intend to stop treating patients until I physically can't anymore. So, unless you sell your practice or move far away from your original clinic location, the sneezers and their referrals will follow you. I still have patients who remember when I started out at my home practice twenty-seven years ago. They remember when they could hear our children screaming, fighting and playing in our house.

Ask yourself this,

> **Can I afford not to do everything I can to convert that lead into a lifelong customer and sneezer?**

Can anyone in business afford to lose $10,625?

TAKE ACTION

Work out your figures and discuss them with your associates, staff members, business partners and colleagues. Think about the unique characteristics of your top fifty patients. What do they have in common? Is it age group, income levels, gender, sport/hobbies, location?

Once you figure this out, and it may, of course, be a combination of variables rather than just one, you will have worked out your fan base. It's much easier to find more fans like these than shooting for anyone and everyone.

The income generated from your patients is only a tiny part of the return created by lifetime patients; it's a much richer reward than just the commodity of money or income generation. Of course, you need to operate a sustainable business to feed yourself and your family, educate your children, have a roof over your head and so on. The bigger picture that overrides income is that every one of those patients will be part of your very make-up. They will shape you, teach you, test and challenge you, look after you, make you smile, fill your life with constant gratitude, fascinating stories and, most importantly, a sense of purpose.

Two-way street

YOUR BELIEF IN THE ROLE YOU PLAY as a healthcare professional must never be too narrow or restricted. This constraining mentality is the opposite of how you should think about your role. The part you play is much more than solely to provide treatment, advice or opinion to your patients. It's not just about you. The most significant rewards come to those who give the greatest. Giving unconditionally, not because you get paid, thanked or praised, just because you want to help others and the community they live in is a much broader and expansive mindset that brings extraordinary benefits.

Having the view that it is, in fact, your patients who will give you much more than you could ever offer or deliver removes the ego-mind and allows humility and modesty to prevail. A good test to check your mindset is to ask yourself this question: Would I work for nothing if I didn't have to earn money to live?

Patients will establish a long-lasting association between your treatment and the relief of their presenting symptoms, now and on every subsequent occasion. So, every time they experience discomfort or pain, they associate relief of their symptoms with you and your skills. They will develop an unparalleled degree of trust in you and your business. They will refer other leads to you and your clinic, which allows you to convert them into other lifelong patients. They literally become walking, talking billboards for you and your practice.

Every new and repeat consultation is an opportunity for many things, two-way opportunities, not just for you, but for your patients and their connections. Who wouldn't want that?

Lifelong partners

ONE OF THE MOST INCREDIBLE OPPORTUNITIES you have as a therapist is to educate your patient about their health and treatment, the services you provide, the services your practice offers, and their role in managing their health. Remember, your expectations will become those of your patient. If you think that a new patient is only asking for your help for this episode of symptoms, then that's precisely what will happen.

Use the new patient consultation as an opportunity to educate your patient about the benefits of your treatment and showcase your expertise so they can fully appreciate and understand your true value. It's up to you to educate your patients; it's not up to them to find out about you and what you can do for them. If you don't give your patients what they're looking for, they will go somewhere else, where someone else will readily and happily take your place.

That practitioner who takes your place is like the passer-by who looks down and finds a priceless piece of jewellery on the pavement. They can't believe that someone wouldn't have taken care of this expensive and valuable treasure. They pick it up and make it their own. Not only do they make it their own, but they go above and beyond, not because they need to, but because it's so easy; it's so much easier to be the second therapist and convince someone you can help them when others have failed before you. Of course, as the second or even third therapist in line, you will benefit greatly from hindsight. The results are already in of what didn't work in the past, all you have to do is ask the right questions and you've already increased the likelihood of greater success. So remember, if you drop the ball, someone will pick it up and keep running.

When a patient meets a practitioner who looks after them, who treats them as a lifelong patient and is a partner in their health and wellbeing, they'll look back and ask,

❝ Why didn't anyone else help me like this before? ❞

Systems and processes

ALL SUCCESSFUL BUSINESSES have a system for everything they do. The system and inherent processes within that system become the way they do it at that business.

In a health clinic, that might be the way you prepare the patient for the consultation, the way your reception staff greet the patients, the welcome that practitioners offer, the dress code, the questions that are asked as part of the new patient onboarding form, the cancellation or missed appointment policy. It's the clinic system that is applied to every patient experience. Failure to apply a system leads to disorder, random results, inconsistency and chaos. It's a hit-and-miss approach that may even lead to patient complaints or, even worse, an adverse event.

It's important to remember that having systems and processes in your healthcare business is not just about checklists or making sure you do specific tasks. Anyone can complete a list or fill in a form. *How* you do things and *how* you say something is of much greater importance than simply completing the steps that make up a system. Your attitude, emphasis, and the order in which you say something, even how you move, are essential ingredients of every successful patient appointment.

The more we say or do something, the more confident we become at saying and doing that action. We take on a sense of leadership, reliability, structure and foundation of knowledge in what we are doing and saying. In the same way that you have a system for examining a knee joint or assessing someone's spine, the entire patient consultation becomes a parent system made up of mini systems.

First contact

TECHNOLOGY HAS MOVED SO FAST in the last twenty years that it's challenging to keep up. In a few years or even less, my advice in this section may be out of date; you need to stay current just like you do with the latest journal articles and research. Most clinics now use technology that makes their administration work easier and more efficient. The internet has enabled online booking, cloud-based patient record-keeping software, desktop and mobile-friendly websites, email and SMS appointment reminders in our healthcare businesses. These advents have undoubtedly been helpful for many therapists who are keen to offer the services that patients now expect.

One of the latest ways that I use and recommend for welcoming and greeting patients before they even arrive at the practice is to send them a thirty-second video message. Many subscription services allow you to record a welcome clip, which can then be texted or emailed to your patient before their first visit. I use Bonjoro, which is easy to use; it's an inexpensive must-have subscription. These short greeting video clips can be sent to patients before they attend for the first time and when they make an appointment for a new problem. This unique approach is a great way for you to distinguish yourself from others and have your patients talk about this wonderful message their therapist sent to their phone.

Video is becoming the new communication medium; it's taken the place of email. Emails suffer from low open rates, high spam detection and subsequent burial in never-opened junk folders, diversion filters and, even if they do make it into your inbox, they sometimes get missed or just become part of your growing unread list.

Very few people read their emails every day. This is especially true if you're not expecting an email, and patients won't be expecting an email from their therapist. The novelty of receiving the video message is part of the surprise. Even if you explain to your patient that they should expect an email in their inbox once they make their appointment, that means they have to remember to check their email inbox. People seldom have email notifications on their phone or laptop unless they are in business.

Think about this yourself. Are you more likely to read something sent to you by email or something that arrives on your phone as a text message? Of course, it's your phone. We can't get enough of the things, so much so that most phones these days keep a record of our daily and weekly screen time as a gentle health reminder to all users.

If video is not your thing, then you can always send a text message directly to the patient's phone or call them so you can connect with them. It doesn't really matter. It's the gesture that makes the difference. How the message is conveyed is almost irrelevant.

As part of my education business, I have built a dry needling video training membership site. I use Bonjoro video clips to welcome every new member. My video greeting open rates are impressive, reaching 97 per cent on average, with 67 per cent engagement. Engagement means that your patient can be asked to perform a call to action (CTA) within the video message. A high engagement rate means that lots of recipients will perform the action you asked them to do. The following is a new patient script, that is based on my membership site messaging, the CTA in this example asks them to click the link, which is part of the message.

> Hi Susan, it's Luke from the Sports and Spinal Group in Hampton. Great to hear that you've made an appointment with me at 2 pm on Thursday, next week. I'm really looking forward to helping you with your back problem. Just one thing to make life really easy for you, make sure you click the link at the bottom of this video. It will take you to our website. Please complete the health questionnaire before you come so we can make the most of your appointment and get you back to function quickly.

Of course, this is only an example; you can vary your script to suit your patient and what you'd like them to do, or CTA, after watching your video message. However, you word your personalised video message, it must always make use of the engagement opportunity by including a CTA. That is the whole point of the video message.

The CTA is at the end of your message because that's the best place for an action that you want someone to remember, never at the start or the middle.

The action you'd like your prospective patient to do could be any number of things, including completing a health questionnaire, remembering to bring their private health fund card, and relevant scan results or referrals; or it might be an opportunity for you to present information about your clinic's services before the face-to-face appointment.

The page where you send your patient to perform the CTA is known as the 'landing page'. An essential function of a landing page is that it must be relevant. It must speak to your lead and transform them into a prospect. They must feel that you've listened to them. You have paid attention. You've made this page just for them. It's a customised tool that kick-starts your lifelong relationship with this lead.

The business process is very much like a dance. Initially, the lead makes their move in response to yours. Once they click on the desired link, make an appointment or complete an onboarding form, they become a prospect, and the dance continues, one move at a time. Your job is not to step on their feet.

It's effortless for your reception staff or yourself to ask a simple question about your prospect's primary complaint on their first contact with your clinic.

> Can you help me by explaining where your primary area of pain or discomfort is located? Is it your lower back, neck or something else?

It's that easy. You can then use this information to make your communication highly relevant.

You now have the full deck of key pieces of information you need to communicate with your client using targeted and tailor-made relevancy, all before they've set a foot in your clinic. Your welcome video message greeted them using their first name, referred to their appointment time and included mention of their primary area of complaint. Once they watch the video, trust builds, but it doesn't stop there.

Relevancy is the most important ingredient in all communication, especially when you're in sales. Using the information that your prospect has given you in order to refine your message is essential. The information on your landing page can also be customised to suit your prospective patient.

Imagine your lead arrives on your landing page and is greeted with:

> Thank you, John. I'm looking forward to welcoming you to our clinic at 2 pm on Thursday 2nd May 2022, and a small thumbnail image of you.
>
> I've prepared some great information about the most common causes of back pain, what we can do to help and the research evidence behind our treatment approach. Please click here to read this information or download it to your device. Please don't hesitate to contact me if you have any questions that you'd like to ask before your appointment.
>
> Emma Smith, Senior Physiotherapist

Your landing page could be used to allow your prospect to upload previous scans to your secure server, complete a health questionnaire, change their appointment time or set reminders for their appointment. This type of landing page would take no more than sixty minutes to design and another sixty to build. You can get an IT specialist to arrange hosting, create a domain-specific email address and even create your unique social media handles for as little as US$5 an hour on fiverr.com. The plugins required to customise it with your patient's details are easy to install and freely available. Your onboarding process shouldn't be an extra – it's a must-have for anyone serious about looking after their leads, prospects and customers.

Domains are very cheap and easily accessible through many online stores. Once you choose your domain, make sure you buy all the similar variants so no one else can buy these and confuse your audience. So, if you buy ifixbax.com, you should also buy ifixbax.com.au, ifixbax.online and ifixbax.store. You might also buy the domain ifixbacks because that is too close to the correctly spelt version.

While we're on the subject of domains, don't use a free email provider for your work or business email. The use of free email providers for your email communication is lazy and unprofessional. Using @gmail, @yahoo, @outlook, @me, or @hotmail is generic and does nothing for your brand. You are effectively advertising someone else's company rather than using the opportunity to promote your own. Buy your domain name based on your business name, your name or the skills that you have.

> **TAKE ACTION**
>
> Create your own video, text or phone script based on your own clinic. Road test the message on your colleagues then, more importantly, on your family and friends. They'll tell you what they really think. By creating a touchpoint with your patient before they even arrive at your clinic, you're already starting to build a trusting relationship and setting yourself apart.

At the time of writing, Bonjoro, the company I use for all my video greetings, is offering a special deal. Visit **twohandsgamechanger.com** for more details.

Your greatest asset

MOST CLINIC OWNERS PROVIDE VERY LITTLE in the way of training to their most significant asset, the first person that your patient or client meets in person. Receptionists are given more training in how to reconcile the daily payments, order supplies and how to operate the computer programs used by the clinic than how to greet the gold that walks in the door every day of the week. That makes no sense at all.

I've been lucky in my clinic to have had great receptionists who know me better than I know myself. I've also made some bad hiring mistakes, which I quickly learnt from. I'll go into these mistakes later but, suffice to say, never hire on ability alone. There's a well-known heuristic that advises employers to hire slow and fire fast. I agree with the latter but not the former. In June 2011, I hired Lillian as a receptionist in my clinic, less than five minutes into her interview at the cafe next door. She started work on the same day. You can't pass up exceptional individuals like Lillian, who has continued to be a vital part of the business even after I sold it a few years later. Her sharp mind, keen intellect and excellent organisational skills have positioned her as a key member of the reception staff team.

Another receptionist who has an entirely different skill set is Kate. Kate, a long-time family friend, started as my first-ever receptionist. All I need to tell you about Kate for you to understand her value is that patients come into the clinic just to talk to her, even if they don't have an appointment. They say no one is indispensable, but I would find both Lillian and Kate impossible to replace if I still owned the business.

Like new graduates, new reception staff are left to figure out how to speak to patients, answer frequently asked questions, open and close a conversation with a patient, resolve complaints and prioritise patient bookings. Receptionists have different amounts of experience and training. Your receptionist may be new to this type of work or your clinic. Often, receptionists are part-time and, understandably, providing every patient who walks into your clinic with a memorable experience may not be top of their priority list. Still, it has to be at the top of your priority list because, rightly, the buck stops with you, not them.

The priority level that your receptionists allocate to the patient 'Welcome' is directly proportional to the importance you, as the business owner, give it. If you don't think it's that important, they certainly won't, why would they? If you don't even discuss the 'Welcome' with them, how will they know what to say?

The 'Welcome' applies equally to you as an associate or an employee in someone else's clinic. If you think that this input doesn't apply to you because it's not your business, then you're wrong. It has *everything* to do with you. Whatever your role or contractual arrangements are, you need to have an owner's perspective and approach. Even if you're a salaried employee, it's your responsibility. You are operating a business within a business. The follow-on effects of a weak 'Welcome' are too dire to contemplate.

One way to train your reception staff is to use a script as a framework of understanding between you and the front desk staff. They don't have to learn the lines verbatim, but they need to focus on the keywords, language and messaging. The receptionist's greeting is just as important, if not more important, than your own. You need to ensure that your receptionists are trained to greet your patients in a way that you want your business to be represented. They represent your brand.

All healthcare clinics need a reception staff induction program that trains reception staff in how you want them to do things your way, not the way they did it at the last clinic that they worked at, not the way the other receptionists told them to do it or how they think it should be done. It must be your way.

The training you provide your reception staff and associates should be documented. This will provide clarity, transparency and simplicity about your expectations. For sure, if you leave the reception 'Welcome' up to the staff member and then realise that you don't like it, you'll find it difficult to undo old habits.

Some of the best advice I've ever received about reception staff training came from Australian physiotherapist, entrepreneur and business owner Paul Wright, the Million Dollar Health Professional. Paul's unique communication approach strips away the noise and focuses on the clear signal of your message to your staff, associates and patients. I interviewed Paul on my podcast channel in 2015. I loved the advice he gave about scripts. He said they could make or break your business. He was right!

I attended one of Paul's courses when he first started out as a business coach for healthcare professionals. He asked the audience what their receptionist should say when a patient rings and asks, "Hello, how much do you charge?"

The audience, who was made up of mostly clinic owners, were stumped. As usual, Paul had the perfect answer, "Why, what have you done?" This was genius. Of course, I, along with everyone in the room, wrote the answer down and promptly listened to the 'why'. Paul explained that the person asking about the price of your service was not actually asking about the price at all. What they were asking for was help. The real question they were asking was, "Can you help me?"

He then explained how we often misunderstand our patients because we are highly trained in rational and logical thinking. We think that A always means B, never C. Just like the patient who walks into your clinic and explains that their problem is chronic lower back pain. You will automatically focus on the back pain, but that's not their problem. Their real problem is what the back pain is preventing them from doing. By focusing on the emotional reasons behind your patient's questions, we provide much more relevant answers. You can find out more about Paul Wright and how he can help you as a clinic owner or a therapist on my website (**twohandsgamechanger.com**).

In the end, how your front desk staff are trained to greet your patients is really up to you or the clinic owner. Naturally, your receptionists should provide every patient with excellent customer service, which begins with a warm and friendly greeting, but what does that mean?

How do we make a greeting so memorable that every patient who comes through your clinic door feels comfortable and at ease every time? Here are some ideas that should help you create your reception greeting script, systems and training. As soon as a new patient walks through your front door, the receptionist stops whatever they're doing, stands up and smiles to greet the patient:

> **Hello, you must be Mr Richards. Welcome to the Sports & Spinal Group.**

The patient will immediately appreciate they've been noticed and acknowledged; they will feel unique, valued and important straight away. This may seem a little 'over the top' to stop and stand up, but when was the last time anyone greeted you like that? The gesture of standing up and greeting your new patients immediately sends a message to them,

> **You're a valued customer to our business; you're important, we are here to help you and make you feel welcome.**

The full script depends on the circumstances but the essential, no excuses message that must be relayed is, "Hello, you must be Mr Richards. Welcome to the Sports & Spinal Group."

What if the receptionist is on the phone or talking to another patient at the desk? Of course, there are situations when we need to adapt our script. The main point here, though, is that even if your receptionist is on the phone or talking to another patient, they must try their best to acknowledge and give priority to the new patient who's just walked through the door. They might need to put another person on hold or briefly excuse themselves from speaking with another person at the desk. This is an art and skill in itself and only comes from prior training, role-play, understanding and experience of interactive situations when dealing with customers. Of course, a friendly greeting and excellent customer service also apply to any returning patients, but their greeting will be slightly more familiar.

Doesn't it drive you crazy when you walk into a shop and, as you approach a group of assistants who are talking together, they continue their conversation, even though you're waiting for their help? This all-too-common experience is all that it takes to make you, the customer, feel like they couldn't care less about you or the business they work in.

Engage early

WHY IS THE MILK ALWAYS AT THE BACK CORNER of a supermarket? The clear and obvious answer is that supermarkets know the value of engagement. We need to learn from them. Positioning the milk in a place that forces the customer to walk through the entire store before buying the milk means, of course, that customers must go past all the other products in the shop before arriving at the fridge full of the milk and all the most popular items bought by customers. It's the supermarket's way of engaging you with products you hadn't thought about or sometimes didn't even know you needed. They know that the majority of customers buy much more than they intended when they go shopping. Who hasn't gone out to get milk and come back with two or more bags, full of other items they never planned to buy?

Engage new patients by asking them to attend 5–10 minutes earlier than their scheduled appointment time so that they can read and complete any required information before they see their therapist, if they haven't already completed a form on a secure landing page, which they are directed to when they make their initial appointment.

The landing page should be used to make your brand statement and initiate the engagement process. Completing a form that asks them for their address, date of birth, Medicare number, doctor's name, contact phone number or even to mark their presenting area of pain is actually irrelevant to the patient. However, suppose they are asked to provide you with these details, which are only important to you, while they're exposed to your services, skills, experience and other trust-building information at the same time?

A digital induction page presented on an iPad or tablet is ideal for welcoming a patient and exposing them to the services you have to offer and the rest of your team. I can't tell you how many times I have heard a patient say, "I didn't know you had a massage therapist here!" When patients make an appointment with you, don't make assumptions about their knowledge of your business. They will know very little about who else and what else is available.

Another option is to provide patients with a QR code that links them back to your website landing page to complete any information you need on their phone rather than using the old-fashioned and predictable sheet of A4 strapped to a plastic clipboard.

While your patient completes the important information you need, they might also be interested to know that you offer Pilates, yoga, dry needling, massage, acupuncture, physio, osteo, chiro, exercise rehab, naturopathy, a range of nutritional products, pillows, wheat bags and home exercise equipment. At the very least, they should be prompted to opt-in to your regular bite-size message about what you can do to keep them healthy, sent directly to their phone.

Opening ceremony

THE ORCHESTRATED CHOREOGRAPHY begins when you meet your new patient, and it continues until your patient leaves the clinic. You are the conductor of the choreography; you know all your lines and every move.

As Heston Blumenthal, Head Chef and owner of what was the most expensive restaurant in Australia, says, "Service is more important than the food". Heston opened his restaurant, Dinner by Heston in Melbourne, in 2015 and closed its doors in February 2020. Perhaps appropriately, the restaurant doors shut for the last time on Valentine's Day as the love affair with its food sadly ended.

Similarly, everything involved in delivering a patient consultation, even the interactions that happen before a patient visits your clinic, are much more important than your actual hands-on treatment. Seems pretty obvious, but how many times have you been to a practitioner when they call out your name in the waiting room from a distance and never introduce themselves? This conveys a subtle arrogance, which can be so easily avoided by simply introducing yourself.

Watch how your colleagues greet new and repeat patients; you'll be surprised at the range of techniques. Calling them techniques is a little too generous because the problem with many greetings is they haven't been given any thought or due respect, let alone any form of training. When I trained new graduates as part of their internship, we practised this critical skill until they were comfortable with it, and they could walk away knowing if they were the patient, they would be happy to be on the receiving end. The goal was never to copy my greeting. That's important to note. The greeting must be unique to the person offering it.

Here are a few introductions you may like to use:

> Hi Jean, I'm Alice. Welcome to our clinic. I'll be looking after you today.

> Karim? Hi, I'm Robert. Welcome to our clinic. I'm one of the massage therapists here, and I'll be taking care of you today.

> Hi, you must be Jaime. I'm Sara. I'm a sports physio. Welcome to the Sports & Spinal Group. I'm looking forward to helping you today.

In every one of these examples, the patient will feel an immediate point of difference from anywhere else they've been to before. They will feel looked after before you've even started treating them. Trust levels begin to rise before you've even entered the treatment room.

When greeting the patient, make sure that you walk towards them first and get closer before delivering the greeting. Avoid calling out their name from the other end of the waiting room. I've seen this happen so many times when I go to my GP. I'm sure they're unaware of how it looks to everyone in the waiting room because if they did, they would be horrified. To the observer, this cold and impersonal welcome appears as though the practitioner can't be bothered to walk any further than they have to, preferring instead to use their voice and force you, the customer, to walk to them.

Show your patients respect and kindness by approaching them so that they feel important and welcomed, at about the same distance as you would stand if you were about to shake their hand. Make good eye contact and smile. These elements are vital, especially when meeting your patient for the very first time. Instant eye contact shows that you are switched on and interested in them. They need to see you smile to make a connection; so, don't forget this vital gesture, even if they are the last patient of the day.

You will, of course, know the names of your new patients before you walk out to greet them. You will also see the name of your next return patient on your list, but do you know the name of one of your patients who's in the waiting room, who couldn't get an appointment with you, and is waiting to see one of your colleagues? Failing to recognise a patient, especially one who raves about you to all their family and friends, can be embarrassing. This is why it's essential to know who is in the waiting room, not just who is waiting to see you.

Even if they're not your patient, never walk past anyone waiting in your clinic waiting room or coming out of another treatment room without acknowledging them in some way, a smile or a hello. It's just good manners, and good manners are the way you do things at your practice.

Body language

TOO OFTEN, THERAPISTS WALK UP TO A PATIENT looking anxious. This is often due to inexperience and work-related performance anxiety. Your body language is a non-verbal signal, affirming that you're in control, you know what you're doing, and you're going to try to help your patient. You need to project confidence and self-esteem, without being fake or unnatural.

Look at how you walk up to the new patient, the speed at which you walk towards them, the posture you hold and the tone of your address to them. Your posture should be neither too strong or overpowering, nor too weak, with your shoulders dropped and your head looking down – this gives an impression of poor self-confidence.

Walking too slowly towards the patient gives the impression that you have all the time in the world, and you have had nothing else to do all day. Walking too quickly gives the uncomfortable impression that you're in a hurry, and this appointment may have to be rushed. You need to walk at a pace to indicate that you've been busy all day, but you're not rushing to the finish line. Practise your body language with someone who will tell you the truth about how you come across. With almost all this advice and information, role-play is by far the best way to practise. After all, you know what they say:

> Perfect practice makes perfect.

Remember, the more unique the way you do or say things to your customers, the more you differentiate yourself from the pack. It raises you from mediocrity to excellence. So, there you have it: your patient greeting.

What an excellent start: a personalised greeting, a smile, eye contact and great body language. Now let's lead your patient into the treatment room. That's right – you need to lead the way.

Perfect practice

I HAVE ALREADY USED THE PHRASE, 'perfect practice makes perfect'. It's important to reflect on the nuance of this phrase in comparison to the more commonly known proverb, 'practice makes perfect'.

The problem with 'practice 'alone is that you tend to end up repeating the same mistakes if you just keep practising the same skills, over and over again. A better approach might be to clearly identify your goal, then list the steps you need to take to achieve that goal.

Let's take an example that's related to manual therapy. You might be a manual therapist who sees a lot of patients or clients who present with lower back pain. Your goal is to prolong your career by developing a massage technique that reduces the load on your hands, wrists, elbows and shoulder joints. By reducing the load on these joints, you feel less tired at the end of the day, and you can provide a better treatment to your patients.

Once you have your goal you now need to list the steps that will help you achieve the perfect massage technique. You might like to find these by researching the most experienced therapists in your profession and watching them work. You can then decide on the most important components of the techniques they use. If they are experienced, that means they must have been performing the skills that you're interested in for a long time, without significant injury. If possible, ask that therapist to give you feedback on your technique.

An experienced manual therapist is the most likely person to instantly pick up on the poor posture, weight transfer, excessive loading or other biomechanical friction points. Watching anyone who is a world-class performer in any field, you will observe that their movements are effortless. Like a Rodger Federer backhand, there's no extra movement, no excessive loads, not a single bead of sweat; it's breathtaking to watch.

This performance, like yours in the treatment room, can only come through hours of practice on the right things, not just hours of meaningless repetition.

To become a master of your craft, you must focus only on what is hard, not what is easy. The endless pursuit of perfect practice will eventually pay dividends in the form of perfect delivery of your manual therapy skills.

Ready?

YOUR TREATMENT ROOM IS THE STAGE on which you perform your finest work, a showcase of who you are and what you do. Before you invite a patient into your theatre you need to make sure that your show is ready. Let's have a look at room preparation.

It's vital to make sure that you are ready to receive your patient into your treatment room. One of the most frequent patient complaints to registration boards is regarding poor levels of hygiene and cleanliness. Ask yourself the following questions every time you're about to take another patient into your treatment room.

» Would I lie on that table?

» Would I sit on that chair?

» Would I put my face in that face hole?

» Would I walk on that floor with my bare feet?

» Would I put my head on that pillow?

» Would I want that towel against my skin?

If the answer is NO to any of these questions, you need to do something about it. This crucial part of the consultation is often overlooked because we think that the patient won't notice. The scary thing is that patients will see, but they won't tell you. They won't tell you about the strand of hair they noticed on the pillow. They won't tell you that they saw the last patients' make-up encrusted on the face hole as they were asked to lie face down against it. They won't tell you that they felt the wetness of the treatment table cover against their skin and wondered if it was the last patient's sweaty body, or you just took it out of the washing machine and put it straight onto your treatment table.

They won't tell you about these shortcomings to your face, but they will make their statement, loud and clear by leaving and never returning. They will tell their husband, their wife, their friends and their workmates ... and you'll never see them or their family and friends again!

The end result of having a strand of dark coloured hair on your nice white pillowcase is that you've just wasted thousands of dollars because you didn't make sure your room looked like the cleaner had just been through it before each patient walks in. What a wasted opportunity!

> **TAKE ACTION**
>
> To give you a taste of how far you need to go, here are a few benchmark practices.

- Never use a creased or torn paper towel on top of the treatment table cover, even if it has just come off the roll. Why? Because a creased paper towel looks like it's been used before, even if you know it hasn't – the stakes are too high.
- It's good practice to wait until a patient has entered the treatment room before wiping the face hole with an alcohol wipe. This sends a message to patients that you take hygiene very seriously, you care about them, and you also care about what they think about you.
- Your room needs to look as if it has come out of a magazine cover, as if you've tidied your room after your last patient, and you've made sure it's immaculate for the 10th time today!
- You've confidently greeted your patient in the waiting room, made eye contact, smiled, and you now lead them to your treatment room.

Who's in charge?

NOW, WHO ENTERS THE TREATMENT ROOM FIRST?

It's far better to stand at the entrance of the room, allowing your patient to enter first, communicating where you would like them to sit as another sign of respect and humility.

And always tell your patient what you want them to do as soon as they enter your treatment room. There's nothing worse for the patient entering your room than having to ask, "Where do you want me to sit?" as they uncomfortably look around at the possible options.

If they ask, "Shall I sit here?" it's too late. They are now subconsciously beginning to wonder who's in charge.

A rod for your own back

A NOTE ABOUT TIME MANAGEMENT.

Punctuality is so important on many levels; it demonstrates respect for your patient's time. Excellent time management should become part of your personal and business brand, always on time, never keeping anyone waiting.

When a patient books an appointment time, it's reasonable for them to expect to be seen on time and for the total duration of the advertised consultation time to be offered. Cutting a patient's consultation time short because you were running late with your last patient is not an acceptable practice and, in time, it will damage your reputation. Don't be fooled; patients know what time they enter and leave your room.

To avoid running late because a patient arrives late, your receptionist needs to confirm whether the patient is happy to continue with a shortened consultation, or whether they would prefer to reschedule. This transparent communication before the start of treatment avoids any uncomfortable misunderstandings. Whether you run a 15-, 30-, 45- or 60-minute list, it's very easy to run overtime. This is an inconvenience to your next patient and creates more work for your receptionist, who should inform other patients that you're running late.

I once upset a tradesman by being five minutes late for a return visit. He gave me a well-earnt slap on the wrist for keeping him waiting. He later explained that a keystone of his building business is timekeeping. This enabled him to stand out among his tardy and often unreliable colleagues in the construction industry. Lesson learnt. Being punctual is a rod that you *want* to build for your own back. We want people to expect us to be on time; therefore, we need a system to ensure this.

Opening line

SO, YOUR PATIENT HAS SAT DOWN in front of you, and we are ready to go. What next? Well, I can tell you what not to say next. Never say, "What have you come in to see us about?" or "How can I help you today?" These opening lines when taking a case history are fatal. They are too vague and too broad. Despite these two lines being the most common starters, using them will have you on the back foot as soon as you finish saying them. Let me explain why.

How we ask questions, and the order in which we ask those questions in the presenting complaint and history sections is critical. Never ask a patient more than one question at a time. Asking, "How can I help you today?" sounds like one question but it's not, it's likely to lead to an avalanche of information that may be relevant and even important but delivered at the wrong time and order. The floodgates will open and you're going to get drenched.

Poorly worded questions also invite a patient to take control of the history-taking process. You might as well swap seats with your patient and have them complete the presenting complaint, using your keyboard and laptop, because now you've handed over control.

By allowing the patient to take control, you will often lose the thread of the story, you might have to ask the same questions again, you may have to reconfirm details, and you will almost certainly miss important information. This is because you haven't stuck to a system. Asking the same question twice is an error that must be avoided. Patients will pick up that you're not listening.

Your opening line must begin with a brief but clear explanation of your plan for today's consultation. The patient then has a general idea of what to expect and how long each part will take. Your opening line should be something like one of the following:

> " We'll go through your history shortly, but before we do that, I'd like you to tell me where you're feeling pain at the moment. "

> **Thanks for coming in today. Before we go through the history of your complaint, please start by telling me where you are sore today.**

> **Okay, we're going to find out why you needed to come in to see me today, but before we get there, can you tell me exactly where you're feeling pain at the moment?**

Use one of these opening lines every time. They will provide you with the information you need at the time you want it. It also sets the scene for who is in charge of this critical information-gathering process. You're asking the questions. They're answering only the questions that you ask, nothing more. It's the most efficient way of completing the case history.

By combining the settler statement about how you will ask about their history and everything that's led up to this point, you've allayed their fears about not being heard. Getting the tone and word order correct will instantly relax your patient. Their shoulders will physically drop when they realise that you're going to listen to the whole story.

Many patients will naturally want to tell you their story, the story that led them to you. You are also interested in their story but not in the way they want to recall it. Your job is to deconstruct their story into useful and ordered information that will help shape your clinical reasoning process. You need their story recounted in the order that will help you deliver on your mutual goal – the goal to restore their ability to walk, sit, stand, bend, lift, run, sleep, lie, raise or jump. By restoring this return to function, you enable a return to sport, work, travel, play and life. The follow-up question about their pain site is the prompt they need to provide you with your first line in any case history. The first line should look like this:

Pt. c/o constant/intermittent, dull ache/sharp pain over the R-CLB radiating into the R buttock and occasionally into the posterior thigh up to the post. knee. No s/m phenomenon. 3-7/10.

This information is an important initial reference point, not only for you, but anyone who reads the notes subsequently.

Use closed questions throughout the entire history-taking process; otherwise, you will relinquish control. You don't have time to veer off-track. If you want to get the job done efficiently and accurately, use a system of questions asking the patient relevant, clear, concise and targeted questions.

In a thirty-minute new patient appointment, the case history should take no longer than seven minutes, less if the patient has completed an online health questionnaire. This leaves you with less than twenty minutes to examine and treat your patient; there's not much time for fluffing your lines.

TAKE ACTION

Record your opening line and the dialogue that follows next time you see a new patient. Listening to your recording may surprise you. Pay attention not only to what you say, but how your patient responds. Compare what they say and how much of that information is helpful in the context of your history-taking process. Think about more efficient ways to extract the information you need using precise language and word order. Before pressing record on your phone, you should, of course, ask permission from your patient. Let them know that you're conducting research about the best way to complete a history.

The *sine qua non* or essential condition of writing includes the three words: accuracy, brevity and clarity. As Dr David A. E. Shephard, MB, FRCP(C), Scientific Editor of the *Canadian Medical Association Journal*, wrote:

> There can be no shortcuts if one is to be sure of conveying one's message so that it is received, one must be clear. Clear thinking, a logical approach to organisation, choice of the right word, relationships of sentences to each other, and paragraphs to each other are the keys to clarity. Still, to achieve clarity, one must be motivated to write well. Rules, then, are most helpful, but help is required in their application.

What happened next?

ONCE YOU'VE COMPLETED THE SINGLE SENTENCE that describes your patient's presenting complaint, you'll need to detail the onset and then the history.

The presenting complaint, onset and history are intervals that can be plotted along a timeline. The start of the timeline is on the left of the page and represents now. This interval denotes the patient's current symptoms. Everything to the right of this point is what happened before they visited your clinic. The first interval immediately after and to the right side of their presenting complaint is called the 'onset', sometimes referred to as 'recent history'. This period should detail the lead-up to the presenting symptoms.

The onset is the detail when their symptoms began only on this occasion and led up to the current presentation. 'Only' is the keyword here. We are *only* interested in this most recent episode. The onset interval may be days, weeks, months or years in the case of chronic pain.

If the present symptoms have never happened before and this is a single episode, then the onset is their history. We don't need to go back any further than the start of their onset. If the patient has had more than one episode of the current symptoms, then the history is a different interval distinct from the onset. The history sits to the right of the onset on the timeline. The timeline is a continuum. It should have no gaps. The onset starts when they first experienced their presenting symptoms on this occasion and ends with their presenting symptoms at the time of their consultation. If the patient has had previous episodes of the same symptoms in the past, then there's a history. The history starts when they experienced their current symptoms and ends when the onset commences.

The single question that you should ask throughout the onset and the history to obtain the required information in the most efficient manner is,

❝ What happened next? ❞

By continually asking this question, you'll ensure that you stay on track, follow your patient's story without leaving any important details out of the case history.

You need to start the onset by cueing your patient because what you need to know will not be immediately apparent to them. As soon as the presenting complaint sentence has been completed, you need to explain the next part of the structured process by saying:

> *If we are talking about the most recent episode of your lower back pain, when did it start?*

Notice that I am asking a single question. I am not asking, "When and how did it start?"

Significantly, this sentence order clarifies which episode you're currently interested in rather than another commonly used phrasing, which can be vague and misleading. If, for example, you asked the patient this question: "Tell me when your back pain started", you'd most likely get the answer that you asked for but not the one you want. The patient will most likely start by telling you about the fall they had twenty years ago, which of course, is their history, not the onset. By prefixing the question with "most recent episode", we switch focus to this event, not twenty years ago. My research shows that the use of the prefix sentence, "If we are talking about the most recent episode of your lower back pain", is twice as likely to communicate that I am asking about the recent onset of their current symptoms and not any historical information that dates back to before this interval.

The other important inclusion in this opening line is the reference to the patient's current symptoms. By recalling their symptoms in your question, you will gain the trust of your patient. They begin to feel that you're listening to their story, even if it's not how they might tell the same set of events to a friend over a drink or two.

Once you're on your way and your patient has been positioned at the correct starting point, the information will begin to arrive in the order you need to receive it. Your objective now is to keep them on track. Guiding your patient is achieved by using this simple sentence: "What happened next?" This phrase is used throughout the onset and history sections.

> **TAKE ACTION**
>
> 1 Create your onset opening lines and test them to see if they achieve the results you are looking for.
> 2 Make sure they refer to the patient's current symptoms and remove any unnecessary words.

3 Practise the questions on at least fifty new patients and record the results.
4 Any sentence that you decide to use should contain only one question.

Testing is critical even for this qualitative hypothesis; it will add meaning and confidence to your language.

The shepherd and the flock

THE SECTION AFTER THE ONSET IS THE HISTORY. The history is when they say, twenty years ago, I fell over while I was on a school excursion. At this point, there's a greater chance of losing your way and wasting valuable time, which is why you need to think like a shepherd and their Border Collie, tending the flock of one. You are the shepherd and your words are the Border Collie. Like the energetic herding dog, you'll use carefully constructed sentences posed as questions to guide the metaphorical flock. Your questions will cajole, guide and redirect them towards the pen.

As your new patient veers off course, you gently restore order with a nip and occasional bite, ensuring that you arrive at the pen together. At the end of the history taking, your patient should feel that you've given them enough space to tell you their story and, more importantly, you've listened.

A good history taker will be able to sift the wheat from the chaff. Like a sieve, you'll only retain the relevant information and accurately discard the extraneous chaff.

The final part of a case history includes questions about aggravating and relieving factors, medical health and family history. This part is where you'll need to ask relevant questions about their health in the context of their presentation. It is also the section where many therapists switch off and treat the exercise as though they were completing a checklist, a checklist that applies to no one and everyone, rather than the person in front of them today.

The case history questions about aggravating and relieving factors are an opportunity for the famous Dorothy Dixer questions. Elizabeth Meriwether Gilmer, otherwise known by her pen name, Dorothy Dix, was a well-known 19th-century American feminist, journalist and columnist. Gilmer's legacy was her ability to frame questions that enabled her to give the answers she wanted. This clever method of inquiry led to a widely used expression, 'Dorothy Dixer'.

You will have heard an example of a Dorothy Dixer if you have ever been unfortunate enough to witness the schoolyard antics of our elected representatives during parliament question time in any democracy. A backbench member asks a minister from the same party a question that enables the minister to make a favourable announcement in reply. This rehearsed carry on is thinly veiled and a waste of privilege in a parliamentary setting, but in our treatment rooms, its use yields excellent dividends for the patient, gaining even greater confidence in you as the therapist.

Any experienced practitioner already knows the answers to the questions about the aggravating and relieving factors before the patient answers them. There are patterns and characteristics for all presenting complaints, and histories that follow predictable algorithms.

There is nothing more impressive for a patient when you can tell them what's making their pain worse or better without them telling you in response to your question. Over time, you'll build up connections between specific presentations and their related aggravating and relieving factors with a degree of accuracy proportional to your experience.

It's even more impressive when you remind them about something that aggravates or relieves their symptoms that they'd previously forgotten!

Here are a few Dorothy Dixer examples:

Differential diagnosis: Plantar Fasciopathy

» "It's probably really sore first thing in the morning, is it?"

» "Gets better as you walk around?"

» "Better at the end of the day?"

Differential diagnosis: Suspected Lumbar Radiculopathy

» "Bad, turning over in bed?"

» "How's sitting on a soft couch or sitting at work?"

» "Getting up off the toilet painful?"

Differential diagnosis: Suspected Lateral Epicondylalgia

» "How's shaking hands – painful?"

» "Turning lids, what's that like?"

» "Can't play racquet sports?"

These types of questions are not just unidirectional, not just for your amusement, nor are they solely used to build trust and confidence. The questions arrive back as answers that provide you with essential information about the degree of severity and impact on function and they start to build your closing advice about what to avoid and what to continue doing.

A word of warning. Getting a 'Dixer' wrong can undo everything you've worked hard to build. Don't start guessing what aggravates and relieves your patient's presenting complaint. Your questions must be informed, not stabs in the dark. Egg on your face is inevitable but measured risk-taking is an acceptable strategy because of the disproportionate rewards.

Matching

THE MEDICAL HEALTH SECTION OF THE CASE HISTORY is perhaps the most likely to be deemed irrelevant by the patient.

Not all questions in this category are, however, irrelevant. Only you can decide how to include or reject them. For example, asking a patient who presents with a traumatic lateral epicondylalgia about their bowel and bladder habits is irrelevant.

But asking the same questions of a patient who presents with lower back pain is highly relevant.

You need to be selective. Match your questions according to the answers you've already been given. If you're running out of time or you just think there's no immediate benefit to asking these questions before your examination, why not ask them after you start treating your patient while they're on your table, getting treated?

Think ahead

AT THE END OF THE CASE HISTORY, you should be ready for the patient examination. The examination is a profession-specific process based on several variables, including the scope of practice, speciality and experience.

Like the presenting complaint, onset and history timeline, there should not be any gaps during the examination process. By 'gaps', I mean no awkward silences when your patient is wondering what to say or do. You should not forget your place on stage either; your patient needs to know exactly where to be and what to do, at all times. It should always be a smooth transition to a new scene. This can only be achieved if you stay one step ahead of them. You should find it easy to think ahead because you've attended the rehearsal as part of your training, they haven't.

Once you have completed the case history section, you'll need to explain what happens next. Perhaps something like this:

> Ok, great, we've got all the information we need. What I'd like to do now is examine your lower back so we can find out what's causing your pain. Is that okay with you?

Your first instructions may be about wearing a gown or removing some items of clothing. If you ask them to do either, leave the room and give them space and privacy to get ready. Explain exactly which items of clothing they should remove and why. For example, ask them to remove a T-shirt but leave their bra on because you'd like to examine the spine. Always ask about the room temperature before you leave. You might be quite comfortable at 22 degrees but they're about to remove clothing and may ask you to warm the room up. It's all about them, not you.

Make sure you ask them to do something after they have removed their clothing or worn the gown.

That something could be,

> Once you're ready, please have a seat, just here,

or

> Once you've got the gown on, please lie face down on the treatment table.

Don't make the mistake I made in my first locum back in Epsom, Surrey, UK. I was filling in for a friend who was going on holiday for two weeks. The practice owner had relied on my colleague's recommendation, and I started work immediately. I had back-to-back patients five days a week. It was great to be so busy and learning so much. One afternoon, I had a new patient booked in for an appointment. I took her history, and before I left the room, I said these immortal words: "I'll be back in a minute if you'd like to get ready."

I returned as promised to start the examination and treatment. I walked in to find the 85-year-old woman stark naked, looking straight at me with great expectation. Time stood still as I scrambled for a suitable response that wouldn't embarrass her or me. It was one of those Catch 22 situations where if I had panicked and said, "Oh, can you please put your clothes back on", or if I said nothing at all about her nudity, it could have gone horribly wrong.

I opted for "Right, can I ask you to lie face down on the table?" and politely placed a large towel over her body. All of this because I fluffed my lines. I wasn't clear about my instructions. It was entirely my fault. Getting ready in her mind was to remove all items of clothing.

The clarity of your instructions must be applied throughout the entire examination and treatment process. If you know that you're going to examine their knee next, then tell them straight after the last instruction that you now want them to lie on their back with both knees bent up or legs straight out in front of them. There should never be a pregnant pause during the examination. It should be ordered, systematic and purposeful. Be as specific as possible. Don't get caught out thinking about what to do next.

Place more emphasis on performing the tests and examinations that cause their familiar pain than anything else. Like the Dorothy Dixers earlier, nothing impresses a patient more than finding and reproducing their familiar pain, especially if you can do this without their help. The more experience you have, the more Dixers you can use, just like in the aggravating and relieving factors, without ever becoming suggestive of a preferred answer or response.

Everyone has pet hates. My pet hate is listening to students and therapists when they ask questions like:

» "Is it sore here?"

» "Does this hurt when I press in here?"

» "What about there, painful?"

» "Is that where your pain is?"

» "What happens when I do this?"

These are dreadful questions because they have the effect of completely undermining you. The messaging that these random questions send is that you still don't know anything about the patient's likely aetiology even though you have used half the available consultation time to try and find the cause of their presenting symptoms. The more of these types of questions you ask, the more likely it is that the trust you've built between you and your patient will unravel right before your eyes.

Once again, it's true that an experienced therapist already knows the results of their examination findings, given the history information provided. As a new graduate, though, you need to avoid the lazy and easy option of asking these open questions before they become habits that are hard to drop.

> **TAKE ACTION**
>
> Practise replacing the first question with the second and see if you're right.
>
> "Is it sore here?"
> → "It's sore here, isn't it?"
>
> "What about there?"
> → "It's there, isn't it?"

"Is that where your pain is?"
→ "This is where your pain is, isn't it?"

"What happens when I do this?"
→ "So, if I did this, your pain level increases, right?"

You're still asking questions, but it's how you ask them that changes how the patient perceives you. You'll know when you get this right, when your patient starts asking you how you know where to press, what's going to hurt, what position brings on their familiar pain and which areas have no pain.

Who do you know?

DURING ANY CONSULTATION, not necessarily during the history taking, there are some significant opportunities for you to gain your patient's trust. One of these is the patient's General Practitioner or family doctor. If you know their doctor through any of your other patients or personally, then this is the time to let them know. "Oh, I see your GP is Dr Sheila Phan. She's great, isn't she? I've known Sheila for a long time; she's very thorough." So now you have someone they know and trust already to build their trust in you. If there's a GP connection, you should write to the GP, with your patient's permission, and let them know you're looking after one of their patients.

The person who referred this patient is another networking opportunity. If your new patient was referred by a patient who you have seen in the past, why not say, "Oh, I see Maria Sanchez referred you. How is Maria?" Avoid any details about why Maria came to see you so that you can protect her privacy. However, you can use the fact that Maria referred the new patient to build further trust. Once again, a thank-you letter to the referrer is another networking opportunity.

The delivery method for both of these networking opportunities is another chance to further promote your brand and how you do things. Using email to communicate with the GP of a patient or a client that refers a new patient is likely to result in your efforts languishing in the recipient's spam folder. One way to avoid this is to send a physical letter, yes, a letter in an envelope with a stamp on it. Address the envelope using a pen, resist the temptation to create a sticky label from a printer. You may already be thinking that will take too long but remember the reasons why you should do this. This process is exactly what I did when I set up my first clinic in Bayside, Melbourne in 1994. It worked wonders.

The largest medical clinic in the area contacted me within months of my practice opening and asked us to present to the group of doctors working in the clinic. After our presentation, we literally received a referral a week for years afterwards.

Now you might be thinking about a compromise short-cut, print a letter but write the address by hand. This short cut will achieve the goal for the thank-you letter that you send to the referring patient or client because they will open it themselves. It will not however work if you're sending a thank-you letter to a GP. The GP will probably have a receptionist open your envelope and give the letter to the doctor, losing the knockout punch effect of a real letter and envelope read by the person you want to thank.

Starting at the end

ALMOST EVERY GREAT SYSTEM starts at the end, never at the beginning. Think about any projects you've completed, any goals you've achieved or ambitions you've had. They all start with an end point, then you work out how to meet the goal by going backwards. Look at your own goal to become a manual therapist. You had an ambition to become a physio, osteo, chiro or massage therapist at some point in the past. That was the end point, but it was your starting point.

You had to find out more about the requirements involved in becoming a therapist. You applied to an educational institution, studied the curriculum, passed the exams. Finally, you got your graduation certificate and got to wear a funny hat with the rest of your cohort on graduation day. You achieved your goal, your project or your ambition by starting at the end. You didn't start by thinking it would be a great idea to study anatomy, biomechanics and exercise rehab just on the off-chance that you might one day be interested in becoming a manual therapist instead of an accountant.

Now, let's apply this to our new patient. What is the goal for your new patient? It certainly will not be to tell you their five-year history of back pain, rate their pain levels or answer inane and pointless questions about their bowel and bladder habits. Their goal is to leave your room, having had three essential questions answered.

» **1** What is causing my pain?

» **2** What are you going to do about it?

» **3** How long is it going to take?

These are the three goals for every new patient and, by default, they must be your shared goals. Like all goals, to achieve them, you must start at the end. Let's look at these questions and translate them into technical questions that we must answer.

» 1 "What's causing my pain?"
  translates to:
  → "What is my diagnosis?"

» 2 "What are you going to do about it?"
  translates to:
  → "What's the treatment for this condition?

» 3 "How long is it going to take?"
  translates to:
  → "What is my prognosis?"

The purpose of answering these questions mentally as you proceed through the case history and examination is so that you can perform your finale. As you collect relevant data in the form of information from your patient history, examination and testing, you subconsciously construct the answers to this trio of questions.

The finale

THE IMPORTANCE OF THE FINALE cannot be underestimated. Interestingly, your patient will not expect you to answer these three questions. They will only realise how essential it is to know this information once you've told them the answers. They'll immediately realise that's exactly what they want and need to know.

Without fail, once you conclude with the final answer to the three questions, the mental comfort that your patient will feel is like using the right combination to open a safe. The last click opens the door to your professional relationship with them on this occasion and every repeat event in the future. Nothing will be said, but when you get the delivery right, you'll know you've reached a new level of understanding, trust and connection with your patient.

If you don't deliver on the three questions, whether by using the wrong phrases and clunky messaging or whether what you're saying doesn't make sense, you'll never crack the safe. Your three answers are the end. They're the finale. Your treatment is almost irrelevant, especially at the first new patient consultation. In most cases, I never actually treat a new patient on their first visit. Why? Because I've done my job – the most important job is the finale. Like any outstanding performance, as the final curtain goes down, your patient can't wait to come back to start their treatment next time.

The trio of questions and answers are inseparable, and their order is always constant. Never leave one out and never mix up the order. That said, each answer doesn't carry the same weight of importance. The last response to how long it will take is more important because it relates to getting back to what they love doing or can't do right now. It's the only answer patients will remember. The preceding answers related to the diagnosis and the planned treatment area will be heard in one shell-like and out of the other. All patients have only one question that they want the answer to:

> **When can I get back to sport, work or the gym?**

Everything else that you tell them is warm-up material.

We, not I

THE FOLLOWING SCRIPTS ARE EXAMPLES of a finale. See if you can spot the keyword.

- » "Okay, Grace, what we do at this point in the consultation is answer these three questions for you: What's causing your pain, what are we going to do about it and, finally, how long will it take before you can get back to the gym, which is probably what you're most interested in finding out? Is that okay with you?"

- » "So, you came in today with lower back pain that you've had for the last five years."
  Now, remember when you were standing up, I showed you how you were standing in the mirror and the way your back hollows in at the bottom, but it curves the other way between your shoulder blades?"

- » "The cause of your lower back pain is very stiff joints and tight muscles in this area here. Why have you got stiff joints and tight muscles in your lower back? We usually find that the cause of your type of back pain is the amount of time people sit at their desks without any breaks, which is made worse by the weakness in the core muscles."

- » "We see this problem a lot. And it's something we can help you with. What I'm going to do to help you get out of pain is loosen up the muscles in your lower back, buttock region and hips. I'll also loosen up the joints in the lower back, especially here and here, where it's really stiff."

- » "I would like you to book a total of four treatments, one a week. I'm also going to give you a series of exercises that I'd like you to do every day. These exercises will help your chronic back pain."

> » "Now, of course, you'll want to know when you can get back to the gym, right? I'm confident that we can get you back to weight training six weeks from now. How does that sound to you?"

Notice the use of the word 'we' in my explanation. It's important when talking to patients to use the word 'we' not 'I':

> ❝ … what we normally find causes your type of back pain is the amount of time people sit at their desks ❞

sounds so much better than, "… what I usually find causes your type of back pain is the amount of time people sit at their desks."

> ❝ We see this problem a lot ❞

instead of "I see this problem a lot."

> ❝ … definitely something we can help you with ❞

instead of "definitely something I can help you with."

Used in the proper context, the word 'we' gives you much more credibility than 'I'. Using 'we' instead of 'I' converts your communication style from a single source to the whole of your profession. Next time you visit your family doctor, listen to them using 'we'. You feel that the advice coming from your GP is coming from the entire medical profession, not just your doctor! Having said this, the use of 'I' slowly replaces 'we' as your experience increases, and authority builds. Highly experienced medical professionals, like specialists, use 'we' less frequently. They don't need to.

You've waited months to see the expert in the field; without question, you'll pay more to see them than a regular doctor, and you'll hang on every word of the ten-minute consultation to hear them refer to themselves as 'I'. It's all part of the placebo. Who hasn't heard an orthopaedic surgeon say, "I like to perform this type of surgery for your presentation" or "I prefer to do this type of procedure under a general anaesthetic?"

The closing trio script may change when you have several possibilities about the cause of the patient's symptoms and therefore the plan of action. If you don't have a firm diagnosis, you must still answer the questions by explaining the possible diagnosis and the steps you will take to eliminate the uncertainty. Here's an example of what to say when the aetiology is still uncertain:

> » "Okay, Adam, what we do at this point in the consultation is answer these three questions for you: What's causing your pain, what are we going to do about it and, finally, how long will it take before you can get back to work? Is that okay with you?"

> » "Well. When you came in today with a really sore lower back, you said it started two days ago, after you lifted a heavy box at work. Now, do you remember when you were standing before? I showed you how you were leaning to the left, and I explained that was caused by a lot of muscle spasm. Also, you couldn't bend forward at all. You also told me that your back pain got worse when you sit down and get out of a chair. Right, so far?"

The "Right, so far?" is a little cue to make sure your patient knows you've listened to their story.

> There are two possible causes of your pain. Either your lower back muscles have gone into spasm, or you've got a disc problem.
>
> With your type of symptoms, we find that it's not possible to determine which one of these possibilities is causing your pain without doing an MRI scan of your lower back region.
>
> Because you're in so much pain and you're leaving to go on holiday in four weeks. I recommend we get an MRI of your lower back. That way, we can tell you precisely what's causing your pain and, more importantly, start treating you, knowing exactly what's causing your back pain.

If you were not about to go on holiday in four weeks, there may not be as much urgency, but I know that you want to know now. So, we'll get that MRI sorted out for you today.

I'll start by loosening up the lower back joints that we found were so stiff, then relaxing the muscles we found were tight and finally show you a series of exercises that I would like you to do daily. The treatment will make you feel more comfortable and should give you more movement.

I would like you to book five treatments over the next two weeks so that we can get on top of this pain and give you the best chance of going on your holiday without pain. Once we know the results of the MRI, we will review your treatment program.

TAKE ACTION

At the next opportunity to perform a finale, review the following key points and construct your script.

- Explain the story of how you arrived at your recommendation and opinion.
- Start at the beginning with their presenting symptoms.
- Explain why it hurts when they walk, sit, run, lift etc.
- Always use 'we'.
- Let them know if you can help them.
- Don't use jargon.
- The whole story should make sense; explain the story in a logical, step-by-step manner. For example, "This is how you stand, so this puts pressure on these muscles, which then causes you to become stiff in this area."

A right to know

YOU SHOULD ALWAYS RESPECT the patient's right to know what's going on.

They really want to know:

- » what's causing their pain
- » why it hurts when they do a specific movement
- » what you're going to do to get them better.

Now, they may not remember all these things next week, but that doesn't mean that we don't bother telling them because they are likely to forget. You'll also find that patients will get better more quickly when involved in the plan you have prepared for them.

Listen more than you speak

THE TREATMENT STAGE IN THE CONSULTATION is the most valuable time to learn more about your patient and build a relationship. Whether you decide to treat on the first visit or not, explaining what you're doing to the patient allows you to showcase your passion about what you do, share your knowledge and educate your patient, and it gives you a deeper insight into the patient's presenting complaint.

While you're treating your patient, you may learn that your patient is deeply concerned about their symptoms, that your patient is concerned not only about their symptoms but their weight; they may want advice about diet or their posture; they may want advice about their pillow or bed. They may even ask you about something completely unrelated to their presenting symptoms. If you can't help with this problem, then you'll probably know someone who can as you build your network of health professional contacts.

Towards the end of the treatment, allow time to recap the plan you explained earlier and to show your patient any exercises you have recommended. Many therapists conclude the new patient consultation with a written plan that details the patient's examination findings, test results, includes pretty drawings with hatched pen markings denoting areas of muscle tension and squiggly lines highlighting spinal curves. These written handouts never get read and collect dust together with other equally valuable items on a desk somewhere until one day your patient realises their obsolescence and retires them to the recycling bin.

Don't get me wrong. It's not that I think that a written summary is entirely useless. It's the delivery method that is limited and ineffective. A much more effective and customised delivery platform uses SMS text messaging to remind patients about their future appointments. You can easily add links that take your patient back to your website and the same landing page they visited before their appointment within the same reminders. This landing page can also be set up to address their specific action plan, which you or your reception staff can upload. You can add personalised video, voice, text, PDFs, almost any content format, plus links to your booking page or contact form.

An easy way to maintain relevant and valuable engagement with your patient is to record them on their phone performing exercises that you'd like them to complete at home. This creates a valuable resource for your patient that can be accessed anytime and shared with their family members, spreading the word about your knowledge and expertise. The video can be uploaded to their personalised patient portal together with other important information about your clinic and their treatment plan.

The interaction between you and your patient occurs on a stage. The stage is your clinic or practice. Your patient sits in the front row, watching you, the thespian. During the entire performance, you will be judged, consciously and subconsciously. From the moment you appear 'on stage'. How and what you say, the speed of your words, how good you are at listening, your mental recall of critical dates and facts, your mannerisms, the speed of your movements and gestures, your appearance and your position relative to the audience are all part of the critical treatment room choreography which will determine if the thespian deserves an encore and rave reviews. Get this act right and expect queues at the box office and sell-out crowds.

Contested two

IT TURNS OUT THAT THE MOST DIFFICULT shot in basketball is the contested two. According to Chris Bosh, former professional basketball player, five-time NBA-All Star, US National Team Member, and Gold Medal winner at the Beijing 2008 Olympic Games, the stats never lie.

You will not be surprised to learn that basketball is a game played by numbers, especially in the professional US big leagues. Coaches and players alike plan their strategy by avoiding risk. That's why they don't like the contested two as a scoring option. They've realised that it's difficult to score two points while the opposing defence contests the power forward's scoring attempt inside the arc. The lesson here is that if you want to win (or succeed), you must reduce the risk of losing. This also applies to how and which techniques you use in any given treatment.

I've already mentioned Professor Laurie Hartman, the osteopath who inspired many of my peers by demonstrating how manual therapy is an art and a science. During my training, I watched as he would pick up any joint that you cared to nominate then carefully but precisely guide it towards its physiological barrier.

Like a magic act, he would release the tension in the joint and restore its natural mobility with a gentle impulse, momentarily splicing the opposing joint surfaces in a fraction of a second. Such was the theatre that one would not be surprised if a white dove flew out from his cupped hands as part of a finale, leaving the joint rested and enjoying new-found freedom. He never failed to cavitate a joint that he attempted to manipulate. The reason was that he never tried to gap a joint that he didn't think he could cavitate. Not every joint that we assess wants to play. Some just want to stay where they are; the clever therapists know which to leave alone and which to manipulate. Some joints are a contested two – why risk trying to move them when there are other easier options to score? Professor Hartman had worked this out long ago.

The problem with trying to treat every joint restriction you palpate or, indeed, every tight muscle that you feel is like trying to renovate an old house. If you try and move a beam that's in your way or a wall that's blocking your view, the roof is likely fall in on you. Risk mitigation starts by doing just enough but not too much.

Treat like a ghost, and don't leave your patient with nightmares. The adage, find it, fix it, leave it, is a great reminder not to over-treat. If you're treating a tight muscle, stop at the instant it turns into jelly. If your assessment tells you that you have four cervical joints that are not moving optimally in the cervical spine, work out which one will unlock the others and give you the greatest return.

Never resort to heavy treatment artillery by using more force, longer levers, or a hefty dose of your body weight. Like a Federer backhand, your technique needs to be effortless by applying just enough of all the technique's ingredients. Getting this right means that your patients will receive just the right dosage without undesirable adverse events like post-treatment soreness. Getting this wrong will have your patient report that they're feeling worse than they did when they first came to see you or that they're experiencing new signs and symptoms.

Your ghost-like treatment will leave them in disbelief at how their symptoms vanished without leaving any of your fingerprints.

Don't do this!

IT WOULD BE DISRESPECTFUL and, of course, totally redundant to write a chapter about how you should treat your patients; this is entirely a matter for you, given your respective training and scope of practice. However, I do want to share a list of things that you must never do in a treatment room or clinic, regardless of your profession.

JACK OF ALL TRADES, *MASTER OF NONE*

At the end of every dry needling course, we present at CPD Health Courses, we provide the following advice to all the therapist who are wondering how to implement their newly acquired skills; choose three techniques that you've learned at the course that will help the majority of your patients or clients, make sure that you will use them frequently.

Only practice those three techniques in your first month. Master the techniques and use them at every opportunity, once you feel that you can safely and confidently apply the techniques, add another three the following month. Aim to become a master of a few rather than poor at many. My advice is exactly the same for all newly graduated manual therapists, don't try and become a master at all the techniques and skills you were taught at once. Learn your craft slowly and predictably, don't cut corners, perfect your craft.

TWISTING AND TURNING

Don't ask a patient to move more than three times during your treatment. Patients are not attached to a rotisserie above your treatment table. They are in your treatment room usually because they're in pain or discomfort. Asking them to move from prone to supine, to sitting, then standing doesn't make any sense and is exhausting for the patient. If you ask your patient to move more than three times, you haven't thought through your treatment plan enough.

WATCH ME

Don't ask your patient to mirror your active movements during the examination stage of your consultation. Nothing looks more unprofessional than watching a therapist raising their arms above their head to demonstrate active shoulder abduction in front of their patient and asking the patient to do it simultaneously. You're a manual therapist, not an aerobics instructor. If that's what you do, stop and think about the hundreds of ways you can cue your patient to do precisely what you'd like them to do while barely lifting a finger. Use your words together with the lightest of touches to have them perform any conceivable movement.

NO SYSTEM

Don't aimlessly palpate, searching for the right muscle. Too often, I've seen students and therapists chase pain rather than follow a logical and ordered process of palpation. A patient presents with medial knee pain of muscular origin. You suspect it could be one of three muscles that insert onto the pes anserinus. A systematic elimination process should follow instead of searching for the offending tissue everywhere in the thigh and lower leg. One by one, you should check which of the three muscles is causing the pain, compare the pain levels to the other side, and make the call.

NO PROCESS

Equally frustrating is witnessing a plethora of random orthopaedic or active motion testing rather than a step-by-step and systemised process, determined not by a quota but by the results of each test. If this orthopaedic test is positive, we don't need to do this; we need to do that instead. If this range is reduced, we should not bother with all the remaining ranges just because they exist; we go straight to an orthopaedic test or a combination of movements.

I described this 'don't do' as frustrating to watch. The reality is that it is equally frustrating for the patient. As mentioned before, they don't care how well you can perform a sixty-second neuro exam. They just want to play golf.

QUIET PLEASE

Don't forget the purpose of your treatment. Know when to chat and when to speak. Chatting is great and is an integral part of any treatment, but like a conductor, you must orchestrate the treatment room conversation. You must never lose sight of the treatment goal and forget yourself in endless chatter about your last holiday or what's for dinner tonight.

At appropriate times in the treatment, you will need to interrupt the conversation and bring things to focus and attention. Your patient must feel that you are about to say or do something important, such as providing a treatment progress report, giving your patient an instruction that is necessary for the delivery of a specific technique or asking for feedback about the tone of a muscle that you've just treated. Patients do not come back to see you because they want to hear how your lemon drizzle cake turned out, at least not for long. They are coming to see you for a result.

THANKS, BUT NO THANKS

Don't be afraid that your patients will say, "Thanks, but no thanks." Too often, we are overly worried about losing our patients by saying the wrong thing or giving them advice, we think they don't want to hear. You must back yourself. Your patients are paying you for your professional advice.

Take the example of a patient with an acute injury that requires multiple treatments over the next week. If you need to treat your patient every day, every other day or three times in the next week, say so! Your opinion matters. It matters and your patient needs to hear it. A nagging voice in your head might say, that's too many times in such a short space of time, they won't be able to afford it, or they'll never come back because they might think I'm ripping them off. None of these is a valid reason for not giving your opinion; they're all just stories that you're telling yourself to justify not having to say something you're feeling uncomfortable about.

The problem with your story is that if you don't honestly give your opinion, no matter how many repeat treatments it will involve and they don't get better, guess who they'll blame? You.

Worse still, if they don't improve and go and see someone else who does have the courage of their convictions, that's a double whammy. Word may spread. Always tell it as it is.

The patients I have treated who have been the most grateful are the ones that I have told, "I can't help you." Yes, that's right. Patients want honesty. They don't want to be mucked about by charlatans who say they can help every patient who walks into their clinic, whatever the presentation.

The patients or clients that book in to see us as manual therapists have similar presentations and therefore there's already a degree of selection bias in our customer cohort. This self-selection is why it may seem unlikely that we might come across a patient or client that we cannot help in our clinic. However, this situation is actually a double-edged sword: on the one hand, it's certainly favourable that patients with presentations that we are trained to help naturally seek our treatments, but on the other hand we may become lulled into a false sense of security by believing that this patient presents with just another chronic lower back pain or acute torticollis.

There are generally two groups of patients to whom I have said, "I can't help you." The first group of patients present with conditions or presentations that are outside my scope of practice. Examples of these patients include those who present with medical conditions either in isolation or concurrently with musculoskeletal (MSK) ones.

I remember one such patient who I saw in my first few months as an osteopath. It was when I was working as a locum for the osteopath in Epsom, UK, and was seeing fifty plus patients a week, gaining valuable experience as a young graduate. One morning I had a new patient booked in, a seventy-three-year-old male patient who presented with lower back pain, referral into the right buttock and posterior thigh. Once I had examined him, I explained my concerns about his symptoms and why I would not be treating him. Instead, I asked him to make an appointment with his GP who I would call and brief on the reasons for my referral.

My main concerns were the severity of his lower back pain, no previous history of MSK pain and a change in his urinary frequency, in the context of his age. Three days later, his wife called the clinic and thanked me for sending him to his doctor. She had been nagging him for months. His GP had sent him for scans which showed lumbar spine metastasis, which he had suspected were from a primary malignant prostate tumour. Thankfully, he underwent further testing and medical treatment.

I remember other presentations and reasons which concerned me enough to refer back to the patient's doctor including very high blood pressure, unexplained dizziness, and suspected bone fracture during my days looking after my local football team. These signs or symptoms are in a category of 'I'm not touching you until someone better qualified clears or treats you first'.

The other, less common, group of patients that I have not treated have signs or symptoms that do fall within my scope of practice. The reason I have not treated these patients is because I felt that another more qualified and specialised manual therapist would be better equipped to help the patient. One clear example was a patient that I remember seeing a few years ago who complained of routine MSK signs and symptoms, but I thought they would do much better seeking the help of a specialised pelvic pain manual therapist.

You must stay vigilant for the patient who is outside the scope of your practice because missing them can have graver consequences than not being able to help those within your scope.

NO HIGH FIVE REQUIRED

Don't be a bighead. We are all warned about the inevitable event in which a patient returns feeling either no better or much worse. The latter example, I discussed in the section, 'All ears'. But do you know what to do when a patient comes back feeling much better? In many ways, this is the most challenging of patients. You see, the problem with the much better patient is that it is similar to the predicament of the number one tennis player in the world. There's nowhere for you to go but south. You cannot get better than number one, but you can be knocked off your self-appointed podium. Treat the patient who reports that they are feeling much better with great caution. Treat them like you would a new car, until you're confident that they really are feeling better.

Rather than greeting this admittedly welcome news with great fanfare and high fives all round, your approach should be one of forensic curiosity. That's great to hear that you're feeling better, but tell me, do you mean that your lower back pain and leg pain are better? When did you start to feel better, straight after the last treatment or more recently? Are you still taking pain medication or are you better even without them? Are you still symptom free when you run? Have you returned to work yet? How long have you been able to sit for?

All these questions are essential to ensure that you haven't got carried away with a false positive. Your patient will appreciate your granular approach, which aims to accurately record your patient's progress. This guarded approach is much more professional and will likely lead to a considerable level of respect from your patient. It's so much easier to take the road of self-adulation and cursory interest in how your patient has arrived at this welcome juncture in their treatment plan.

Even after this seemingly counterintuitive inquisition, you do indeed find that your patient is really much better based on all qualitative and quantitative scales, refuse the temptation to bathe in your glory. After all, you've only delivered the goods on time and as promised, nothing more, nothing less. The antidote for the temptation to bask in the sun upon hearing such news is the reminder that you're only as good as your last treatment. Whether you've exceeded expectations is best answered by your patients or clients, not you. That is their prerogative.

STICK TO THE PLAN

Do not reveal all your cards at once. In the course of a six-treatment patient management plan, your patient might be expected to show signs of improvement after two or three treatments. Let's take this as the desired outcome for a given patient. Your patient reports that they are so much better after the midway point. Now what? What you must not do is thank the Lord for your good fortune and tell your patient that they never need to see you again. This short-sighted approach is fraught with risk.

The problem with this abandonment approach is that you haven't proceeded with the plan as promised. Your patient may well be better, but better than what? Perhaps your plan provided some initial stretches for tension in the hamstrings, which have done the job, but now we need to progress to the next part of the plan. The next part may include strengthening, working on secondary areas of dysfunction or developing a long-term exercise routine to avoid recurrence. The time to introduce these new longer-term management strategies is when they feel improvement in the early stages of the plan.

Avoid revealing your plan all at once. The plan must be drip-fed at the times when your patient is most receptive. The script might go something like this:

> Great to see how you've improved in terms of your leg pain so far. This is great. I'd like to spread your treatment out now to two weeks. If you're still feeling improvement, I'll show you some important strengthening exercises that will help you avoid the return of your symptoms. We find that these strengthening exercises are really effective as a long-term strategy for this type of presentation.

Completing the recommended management plan is a much better strategy than allowing your patient to think that it's all over as soon as they feel better. If you thought they needed six treatments then, notwithstanding minor adjustments, you need to see it out. Otherwise, your patient will walk away thinking that you have done your job and that their discharge which you condoned, was the right thing to do. We all know what happens next. Your patient hasn't got any long-term strategy for improving muscle strength, flexibility, joint range or whatever the predisposing factors were, and inevitably they go back to square one. Now what?

DON'T ASK

Don't ask a patient what the drug they're taking is for? Patients expect you to know what a drug is used for. Memorise a list of the most commonly prescribed medications, their uses, their generic names and their brand names. Knowing why someone is taking a particular medication is extremely important. Equally, you must never show a gap in your knowledge regarding something as basic as this. A list of the most commonly prescribed medications, their generic and brand names can be found on my website (**twohandsgamechanger.com**).

MUM'S THE WORD

Don't ever discuss the health of one family member with another. I learnt this lesson a long time ago in the most unexpected of circumstances when I saw one of my patients for a routine lower back check-up. I asked how she had been since last time when she reported that her back pain was feeling great; she now felt pain over the calf. The recent onset of calf pain began after dashing across a busy street two days earlier.

I duly examined her and was suspicious about the aetiology of her new symptoms. I couldn't detect any signs of muscle injury, so I suggested that she make an appointment with her GP for an ultrasound scan to check the possibility of deep vein thrombosis. I treated her lower back and thought nothing more about it until I saw her husband a week later.

As I was exchanging the regulation pleasantries with him, I naturally asked how his wife was. Did she go to the doctor and get the scan? It was at the exact moment that the last word of that sentence left my lips that I knew I was in trouble. The expression on his face told me I had dug a big hole for myself, I jumped right in it without my shovel.

He had no idea about the possible deep vein thrombosis, a recommendation to see the GP or a scan. I changed the subject as quickly as possible and awaited my fate when I next saw his wife. Sure enough, at her next monthly appointment, the conversation began with the following opening salvo, "I've got a bone to pick with you." I stood there, embarrassed and not surprised. I had made a mistake in assuming that married couples share their medical health histories. They don't. I took my medicine and apologised. A great lesson to learn.

The irony of this story was that my patient did go to her GP, who agreed with me and sent her for an ultrasound of the painful calf. A thrombus was found and treatment was initiated, after which she made a speedy recovery.

Don't discuss a patient's story with your family using their name. This may seem obvious, but thanks to social media and the ever-decreasing virtual communities we live in, it's not actually that easy to avoid inadvertently identifying a patient. Avoid having to backpedal by using discretion in your conversations at the dinner table.

LETTING GO

Don't ever say, "See how you go", at the end of a treatment. What does that even mean? It means that you don't have a plan with a start and end. It may also mean that you would prefer that you don't see this patient again because you don't want them to come back next week and tell you, "I'm no better." You must face up to failure; we have all had patients return to see us that are not just no better but even worse than they were before they saw you. Apart from listening more than speaking during one of these encounters, remember that even though the patient might not be any better, they still came back. This means that they still need your help and are even prepared to pay you for it.

REGULAR SERVICING

Always recommend maintenance treatment. I didn't say insist on maintenance treatment, just recommend it. Almost every patient that I have seen would benefit from regular manual therapy. The simple analogies relating to regular dentist treatments and car servicing are useful but rarely necessary. Correctly framed and timed, the conversation about the importance of regularly looking after your musculoskeletal system is readily accepted and agreed to by most. The conversation may go something like this:

> Now, it sounds like you're feeling much better than when I first saw you a few weeks ago, which is great. One of the options we recommend at this point in your recovery is an appointment in one month's time to see how you respond without treatment but continue with your rehab program of stretching and strengthening. How do you feel about that?

By first suggesting an interval of one month rather than saying to a patient, I want to see you every month for the next six months, you are doing two things; the first is that you are testing whether or not the patient or client continues to remain symptom free for the duration of the gap in treatment interval. The second is that you are also finding out their level of interest in attending while they're symptom free. Their level of interest in returning to see you will depend on many things, including how they managed previous episodes of the same pain, financial ability, time available and the influence that their family and friends have on them.

When I recommend maintenance treatment, I usually start with one month and then adjust the interval according to how they respond. If they report that they were symptom free throughout the entire month and I find that their tissues reflect how they feel, I will spread the gaps between treatments to six weeks or two months. If they say that things have been great until a few days before their monthly treatment, I might suggest staying at one-month intervals. My normal range for maintenance treatment is between one and three months.

CONTRACTUAL OBLIGATION

Don't move your 5:30 pm patient, even if you have no patients all afternoon. Once an appointment time is made, it's a contract between you and your patient which should never be broken except in an emergency and never for your convenience. Your patient can call and ask you to reschedule but you never can. If you are the one who calls to reschedule, your patient may wonder why?

- » Do they want to knock off early on Friday night?
- » Have they got no patients booked in before me?
- » I have now been inconvenienced. Why?
- » How important am I to this therapist?

Long John Silver

ONE PIECE OF ADVICE that I constantly give to younger therapists is about the importance of accurate patient treatment notes.

In December 2011, I was paid a surprise visit at my practice in Beaumaris, Victoria. The two investigators were from the Private Health Fund, HCF, and were conducting a routine audit of my patient notes, which I had no idea they could do. They wanted access to the patient treatment notes of fifteen of my patients that I had treated over the past two years who were HCF members. The list of patients they were interested in was sent to my clinic fifteen minutes before they arrived; apparently, this ensured that I could not edit or delete the patient records.

They sat politely in my treatment room and examined all fifteen patient notes. What surprised me the most was that they were not just interested in the treatment dates, and whether they correlated with their records, but they were also interested in the details of my treatment and my management plan.

The process took about thirty minutes, and they thankfully concluded that I had kept excellent patient records that complied with the HCF provider agreement. As they were about to leave, I was curious and asked them how many therapists failed the audit. I was shocked to learn that 50 per cent of therapists fail the audit. The reasons for failing include overservicing, incomplete or missing patient notes, fraud, leakage, padding and cascading. Some of these terms were new to me, which got me thinking. My thinking started me on a journey to learn more about Private Health Fund audits and the consequences of failing them. I found out that failing an audit can lead to derecognition by a health fund depending on the seriousness of the breach. Health funds lose tens of millions of dollars every year due to fraudulent practices by healthcare practitioners.

As I learnt more about the problem facing private health funds, I realised there was an opportunity. If I had no idea about the potential for getting audited, then I was pretty sure that more therapists were also oblivious to this fact. What if I created an online program to help therapists remain compliant with health fund terms and conditions? I contacted HCF to see if this might be helpful and met with their executive team in Sydney, Australia. Over the next few months, I created an online learning module titled, 'The Private Health Fund Compliance Program'. It is now available as part of my membership site: **twitch.cpdhealthcourses.com**

The single most important lesson that I learnt through this experience is captured by one image that pops up every time I write up my patient notes. The scene in my mind depicts me writing my notes with a parrot sitting on my left shoulder. The parrot represents the auditors checking to see if my notes comply with the rules. I have translated that image into the advice I give to anyone who asks me about patient note-taking. Write your notes as if you had to defend what you'd written in a court of law. Just before you click Save, ask yourself,

> Would these notes protect me against anyone who claims that I was negligent or incompetent?

If the answer is yes, click Save.

Consent

THERE'S VERBAL CONSENT and written consent; both are required before treatment. You must have a written consent form which your patient reads and signs, then you sign it before you start treating a new patient. The consent form content depends on your profession, the scope of your practice and the therapeutic modalities you use in your clinic.

My written consent form details the possible adverse events that may arise following treatment. I include the percentage likelihood of these events and reference the source of the information I have provided. I also explain the steps that I have taken to mitigate these risks. The consent form explains your treatment and the inherent risks, however small they might be, and provides your patient with the opportunity to opt out of specific techniques that they are not comfortable with.

The purpose of all consent forms is to adequately inform your patient about the possible side effects of your treatment. My written consent form is provided to all new patients as part of their onboarding process. They are asked to read the information but not to sign it until they have seen me. Before I start taking a history, I ask the new patient if they have any questions about the information they've read. If they have no questions, we both sign the form, which is kept on their records. Every patient must complete this process annually, which reduces the chance that a patient claims that they were unaware of the potential risks should they lodge a claim against you.

Verbal consent is used before specific procedures like manipulation of the spinal facet joints. I have a script that I use each time I apply this technique. I record that I have asked for verbal consent on the patient notes.

TAKE ACTION If you don't have a patient consent form, create one today. It's one of the most important legal documents in any healthcare business. Please don't wait until you get a claim or complaint made against you before realising its significance. A copy of my consent form is included on my website (**twohandsgamechanger.com**).

King of the castle

AFTER READING THE CHAPTERS about the new patient consultation, you should be excused for thinking that I may be suffering from the ubiquitous condition that afflicts many of us in the healthcare field, overconfidence bias. The Swiss author of the book *The Art of Thinking Clearly*, Rolf Dobelli, explains how we are all susceptible to this type of cognitive bias. In a well-known experiment that you can play along with at home, researchers ask a group of randomly selected adults who drive a car a simple question: "Compared to the average person, do you see yourself as an above-average safe car driver or a below-average safe car driver?" The group is asked to raise their hands accordingly. The results for any similar cohort are always the same. Ninety per cent consider themselves above average. This is called the overconfidence bias or effect. This famous experiment should, of course, show a fifty-fifty result because the median score should be in the middle of the driving safety range.

Whichever gender you are, you will not be surprised that men are more prone to overconfidence than women. Optimists and, to a lesser degree, pessimists are also pre-disposed to overconfidence. It should concern us that people are generally more confident than they are accurate. Overconfidence can lead to a phenomenon called 'cognitive dissonance', which is another behavioural problem that we should at least be aware of, even if we cannot avoid it.

We need to understand both overconfidence bias and cognitive dissonance and their insidious effects on our ability to think clearly and logically. Any detriment in your capacity to carefully consider the information before you in a healthcare setting can be catastrophic, leading to highly damaging adverse effects on the health of your patients, colleagues that you work with and your business.

Matthew Syed, the British author of *Black Box Thinking*, a book that I highly recommend, describes how the medical profession is among many vocations affected by cognitive dissonance. Other occupations where cognitive dissonance can have a harmful and even detrimental effect include the occupations in law, aviation, politics and the armed forces. Syed defines cognitive dissonance as spinning the evidence before us to fit our beliefs rather than adapting our beliefs to fit the evidence. Your brain alters the facts to reduce the mental worry and restlessness that ensues when you are presented with challenging circumstances or events. The higher one's position of power or responsibility, the more cognitive dissonance is likely to influence decision-making.

In the section, 'All ears', I explained how I managed a return patient who told me that she's never felt worse after treatment in all her years of coming to the clinic. At the exact moment that your brain registers this sentence, you'll start to evaluate the two choices you have before you. On the one side, there will be indisputable evidence and undeniable facts. On the other is, well, a long river in Egypt, denial.

Initially, your first thoughts after the initial sinking feeling in your stomach are questions filled with doubt like: Is this the end of my career? I wonder if everyone in the clinic knows about this. Will the receptionist who passed on the message tell the other receptionists? Will she make a complaint to my boss? Will she complain to the board about me? What did I write in my notes, or did I write any notes?

In the case of the patient who had never felt worse, the facts were that she really did feel much worse, much worse than she had ever felt before any other treatment. Her feelings cannot be contested or given a value based on my metrics or judgement.

On the other side of the equation, my denial process quickly formed in my mind, and with it, the potential for cognitive dissonance. I say 'the potential' because we do have a choice about which road to follow, the one built on facts or the one built on falsehoods created by the brain's protection mechanism and designed to distance you from reality and consequences.

In my mind I quickly constructed the metaphorical scales, the facts versus falsehoods. The denial process consists of usually bold ad hominem statements designed to protect and cancel out the inconvenient truth: She's eighty years old. What does she expect? Nobody has ever complained about my treatment before. I'm highly experienced. She's so sensitive. Her last therapist told me that she's a massive whinger. Of course, she's going to be worse before she's better. A mental equation is generated. Your decision about which of these opposing views you'll follow determines whether you'll fall prey to cognitive dissonance or rescue yourself in favour of reflection, acceptance, problem-solving and empathy.

As healthcare professionals, we're good at altering facts in our favour, says Dr John D. Banja, Professor and Medical Ethicist at Emory University in Atlanta, Georgia. Dr Banja is the author of *Medical Errors and Medical Narcissism*, in which he states,

> Health professionals are known to be immensely clever at covering up or drawing attention away from an error by the language they use.

We learn how to trick, deceive and use linguistic subterfuge during our academic training. Our status in society in general and our communities further supports our fragile belief systems built on nothing more than our subjective opinions and beliefs rather than the facts and reality.

The first thing you should do is acknowledge that you already suffer from overconfidence bias and cognitive bias. It is not unique to you. Just like pain, sickness, need and desire, it is part of the human condition. Once you accept that you are fallible like everyone else, you can begin to recognise the onset and the conditions that predispose you to these essential behavioural traits. The importance of acknowledgement and then acceptance are the first and crucial first steps to avoiding the possible dangerous outcomes that follow these faulty reasoning processes.

We must continually remind ourselves that we are all in practice, not perfection. When an adverse event occurs, it's almost always an accident, never intentional. All healthcare professionals promise that they will abide by the Hippocratic Oath: *primum non nocere*, that is, 'first, do no harm'. There is a cure. If not a cure, there's at least a possible alternative to faulty reasoning processes like cognitive dissonance.

Be curious

THE ROYAL SOCIETY is the oldest scientific academy in the world and is based in the United Kingdom. It was founded by twelve men who met at Gresham College after a lecture given by Christopher Wren, its resident professor at the time. It is now the Fellowship of more than 1600 of the world's most eminent scientists, promoting excellence in science to benefit humanity.

The Royal Society has played a part in some of the most fundamental, significant and life-changing discoveries in scientific history. Its Latin motto is '*Nullius in verba*', which means 'on the word of no one'. In plain English, it means 'don't believe everything you read', or 'take no one's word for it'. I try and live by this motto every day. I think that now more than at any time in our short history on this planet, we must all become more curious. We need to ask more questions, be sceptical, never take anything at face value, be open-minded, test, scrutinise, go beyond the headlines, and always ask why.

Like the Fellows of The Royal Society, we must all be determined to withstand the increasing control of authoritarian governments, treat the news media as entertainment rather than journalism, avoid being fooled by marketers, read the fine print in the scientific literature and always be the contrarian. We must verify all statements by appealing to facts determined by experiment.

'Curiosity' is the one word that describes the best approach to every patient's presenting symptoms. The next time you are faced with the challenges of managing a patient who is much worse or even no better after their treatment plan, be curious about why rather than falling prey to the dissonance processes that inevitably creep into your thinking and you begin to lay blame at the person who sought your help and advice. In the end, it is up to you: if they are feeling no improvement despite your best efforts, then the facts are that, on this occasion, your best efforts were not good enough.

The next time you incorrectly diagnose a patient's presenting symptoms as caused by facet joint syndrome, then it turns out that they have lumbar spine radiculopathy, be curious about how you missed this presentation. Review the information that led to you making the original diagnosis.

Ask yourself ...

- » If you should have or could have made a different decision based on the facts presented to you at the time.
- » What techniques did I use? Are there better options?
- » If you executed the techniques to the highest possible standards, or could you improve on your therapy delivery.

The next time, the boss refuses to give you a pay rise, even though you've been at the same rate for the last five years, be curious about why this seemingly implausible and unfair decision was made. Is it the fact that your boss does not value your work? Is it because if the boss gave you a pay rise, they would have to give everyone else one too? Is it because you're asking for too much money? Is it because you're in the wrong clinic and you need to move to one that values what you can bring to the table? Pun intended.

The next time you start reading the abstract from a research paper, stop reading it and read the article itself. Be curious about how the subjects were recruited, the confounders, the methodology, whether the results have any external validity, and the p values? In my experience, many papers fail the first few hurdles and need generous amounts of salt to be taken seriously. This is why you must never say 'always' or 'the research says X'. A more accurate appraisal is that either 'we do not know' or 'some research indicates X.'

The next time that you look at your empty appointment list, be curious. Do not wander down the road of cognitive dissonance and start blaming everyone and everything other than you. You are the only one who is responsible for your list. It is not the fact that others in the clinic always get new patients. It is also never any of these reasons: the fees are set too high, it's the wrong location, you're not experienced enough, the reception staff don't like you, the parking around here is terrible. It's not because you are so good that all the patients you have seen are pain-free after one treatment. It's because of you.

In every one of the examples I have given above, the answers lie in being curious about why. You must always ask this question if you want to successfully negotiate the inevitable events and challenges that will punctuate your professional life as a healthcare professional.

Not only does the curious approach tame the dissonant and overconfident mind, but it also leads to learning opportunities. They are only opportunities, not necessarily lessons that are learnt. Sometimes it takes us many opportunities before we even recognise them as lessons to be had and a chance to change our behaviours.

It's a numbers game

BASEBALL IS A GAME PLAYED BETWEEN TWO TEAMS of nine players, each on a field with four white bases laid out in a diamond. There are four bases: home plate, first base, second base and third base. The home plate is where the batter attempts to strike the baseball pitched by the pitcher. Each team takes turns batting and fielding. The winning team is the one that has scored more runs than the other over nine innings.

Anyone who has seen the 2011 American biographical movie, *Moneyball*, based on a true story about the Oakland Athletics baseball team, will know the value of numbers. The film's lead, Brad Pitt, plays the part of Billy Beane, the General Manager of the struggling team.

In 2002, the Oakland As, America's lowest-paid baseball team, began the season with a less than auspicious losing streak of eleven losses in a row. They finished the same season with a twenty-game winning streak. This incredible turnaround is attributed to Beane and his appointment of Peter DePodesta, known as Peter Brand, in the movie.

Peter DePodesta is a Harvard economics graduate and was employed by Beane because of his interest in the quantitative analysis of baseball and, specifically, statistical data about batting, pitching and fielding. Using his training in this emerging area of sports analysis known as sabermetrics, DePodesta scouted players based on their key performance indicators (KPIs) rather than the traditional qualitative skills used by other recruiters like observation, intuition and gut instinct. The novel strategy DePodesta introduced involved selecting players based on their on-base percentage metric (OBP). High OBPs combined with a low appeal rating made these players more attractive to DePodesta and his team. The other benefit in choosing the ugly ducklings of the baseball draft pick pool was that they were much more affordable for a struggling team like the Oakland As.

OBPs are a type of KPI. KPIs play an integral role in every sport that is played at the highest level. Today, players from every sport are analysed for thousands of benchmarks and criteria in addition to qualitative analysis, all under the heading of KPIs. The numbers game is a vital part of every business and every aspect of the world we live in – everything from government inflation and employment projections, scientific research, population studies, epidemiology, meteorology and aviation.

In a healthcare setting, the term KPI is still thought of as an intruder more suited to the corporate world than in the empathetic and caring environment of helping patients. New graduates are perhaps more likely to feel pressured when KPIs are used to assess their performance in their early years while they're still finding their feet. A monthly or even weekly chat about the numbers and what they mean can be quite daunting, especially if you had previously thought that no one was able to tell you what to do or not to do once you had completed your professional training.

The problem is not the KPIs themselves. They are necessary, essential, and a vital source of information for both the therapist and the business they work in. The keyword here is 'business'. All serious healthcare businesses collect figures about sales, expenses, revenue, profits, liabilities, wages and customer numbers. This data provides critical information that helps owners decide the best way to manage their business.

Managing a business is not just the domain of the clinic owner. As mentioned elsewhere in this book, you've already signed up for running a sales business, whatever your role as a healthcare professional. If you are the owner of a healthcare clinic or business, then you need KPIs to track your progress, create strategies, manage staff, and align your focus with your goals and objectives. As a clinic associate, you need different KPIs that will track your performance, chart your progress, and provide feedback about your strengths and weaknesses.

The Austrian management consultant, educator and author, Peter Drucker, is widely accepted as the man who invented modern business management. He wrote thirty-nine books on the subject and is widely regarded as the most significant management thinker of all time. The quote,

> If you can't measure it, you can't improve it,

is attributed to Drucker.

There are many other great quotes attributed to Drucker:

> What gets measured gets managed.

> The best way to predict the future is to create it.

> Culture eats strategy for breakfast.

> Most leaders don't need to learn what to do. They need to learn what to stop.

Consider this scenario: a new graduate has been stuck at an average of 25 per cent of total capacity for the last three months. This means that if the graduate could see a maximum of forty patients per week, they only see ten on average. So, there's a problem that needs addressing.

The challenge is unrelated to the metric itself; that's just a number. The challenge is different for both the clinic owner and the new graduate in this case. Once again, both sides must start at the end. What do we want to achieve at the end of this discussion? Yes, even the new graduate may want to ask themselves if they have been mentored and supported appropriately.

Having a conversation about KPIs with anyone, especially a new graduate, should be handled with sensitivity by the business owner, with clear goals and objectives in place. These boundaries should have been explained as part of the initial induction process so that there are no surprises: this is how we do things here. Correctly framed, both parties should actively welcome the KPI review.

There are many possible KPIs healthcare businesses could use every day. The problem with too many numbers is a bit like the problem with too many questions during the history section of a patient consultation. You end up confused, with a lack of purpose or direction.

I tried to keep things very simple in my practice, extracting only five-weekly KPIs: income by practitioner and therapy, average fill as a percentage of total capacity, total new patient numbers, total patient numbers and the average number of times a new patient returns. If I had to choose just one metric, it would be the average fill as a percentage of total capacity; basically, how full is your list.

All the other metrics are generally derived from this single ratio. If a therapist has a full list most of the time, the KPI chat will be very short. Longer discussions are likely if the list has a lot of white spaces between the bookings. It's really that simple.

In my experience KPIs are very important for the business owner for the day-to-day operations and if the owner ever wanted to sell their business. They are also crucial as a reference point from which to start the conversation with underperforming associates. The only discussions that a business owner needs to have with the therapist who has a full list all the time are about increasing the fees they charge or the opportunity to buy into your business.

If you are the associate with the full list all the time, then don't wait for your laggard boss to have a chat with you. Book that appointment with them today. If they haven't recognised your real potential, you need to present that reality for them, front and centre.

Agree to disagree

OVER THE LAST THIRTY-FIVE YEARS, I have employed or contracted many people, including healthcare professionals, reception staff, cleaners, business managers, bookkeepers, accountants, mentors, graphic designers, vehicle wrappers, virtual assistants, computer programmers, website designers, forum moderators, videographers, copywriters and landing page developers.

I have drawn up different contractual agreements to suit the position that I wish to fill. Some arrangements are straightforward: full- or part-time contracts that do not require much input on my part. Others have been customised over time following a mistake I've made or after learning something new from a course, reading or research. Any well-structured contract aims to mitigate risk and ensure clear communication between the two people signing the agreement.

When I have employed people that require access to my intellectual property, I always use a Non-Disclosure Agreement or NDA. An NDA is a valid legal document that details what you are willing to provide access to and the limitations that you wish to impose. Importantly, it also specifies the consequences of breaching the agreement. A sample copy is included on my website (**twohandsgamechanger.com**).

I've learnt in dealing with people and employment contracts that even if you have the best possible contract written by the best legal team in the world, it will not stop someone from interpreting and perhaps behaving in a way that is contrary to your understanding of what the original terms and conditions were intended to mean. At that point, it will not matter whether you have a signed contract or not. What matters is how deep your pockets are if you want to use a legal team to make your case or how much you're willing to do the work yourself. I have done both: I have employed a legal team to protect my intellectual property on more than one occasion and when I applied for a trademark. I have also overturned a state government statutory authority judgment that threatened to bankrupt me, using my research, letter writing skills, and hundreds of hours after work. I used the same skills and resources when I received a 'please explain' letter from my professional board. The board sent me a letter asking me to respond to a complaint they had received. The essence of the complaint was advertising, explicitly using a photograph that I had placed in my clinic window. The picture was taken in 1985 at the British School of Osteopathy during a visit to the school by none other than HRH Prince Charles. I was in the photograph standing on one side of the next heir to the British Throne, and two other senior students. At the bottom of the picture, I had added the following sentence: Wayne meets HRH Prince Charles.

The inference made by the complainant was that I was using this photograph as a testimonial. My argument was that I was not using this photograph as a testimonial because, in the photograph, he is not seen to be treated, nor was he presented as a patient. I had no choice but to respond to the claims. I was then asked to take down the photograph, which I did. As the cliché goes: you need to pick your battles; that is, weigh up the risks versus benefits while considering the inevitable financial costs and the effects on your mental health.

You may be wondering why I used the name Wayne on the picture I referred to above rather than my real name, Wael. Well, that's because my real name is very difficult to pronounce for non-Arabic speakers. To make life easier for everyone, including me, I started using Wayne soon after I arrived in Australia where first name terms are much more common than in the United Kingdom.

Hiring and firing

I HAVE EMPLOYED MORE THAN ONE HUNDRED PEOPLE and interviewed more than four hundred others to work in my clinics and now in my dry needling education business. The single most important heuristic that I have learnt and the one that guarantees success almost every time is hiring someone you like.

There are no rules about this potentially dangerous but necessary exercise for every business owner. If you get it right, you save yourself so much time. If you get it wrong, you'll create a massive headache for yourself and everyone affected by your decision to hire or fire.

There are more things that you shouldn't do when hiring and firing than things that you should do. I have learnt what not to do from reading hundreds of business books and listening to thousands of podcast episodes. On average, I listen to forty books a year using my Audible App. I love listening to podcasts and books while on a plane, exercising or driving.

One of my favourite podcasts is by Tim Ferriss, American entrepreneur, author and investor. Tim is perhaps best known for his books *The 4-Hour Workweek*, *The 4-Hour Body*, *The 4-Hour Chef*, and *Tools of Titans*, which I mentioned earlier in the section about journaling, and *Tribe of Mentors*.

His first book, *The 4-Hour Workweek*, spent more than four years on *The New York Times* Best Seller list. It has been translated into more than thirty-five languages and has sold more than 2.1 million copies worldwide.

His podcast, *The Tim Ferriss Show*, focuses on deconstructing world-class performers from every area of achievement, including sport, business, health, science and investing. He skilfully draws out habits, stories and rituals and routines from his guests. His podcasts have been downloaded more than six million times, on multiple platforms.

I've learnt some great tips about hiring and firing while listening to Tim and the many polymaths who have been guests on his show. However, I haven't just used the ideas and suggestions straight off the shelf; I have adapted and tested what I've learnt and converted what I've learnt into a valuable library of interview questions and strategies for many different roles in my businesses.

Never ask a lame question like "Tell me your most significant weaknesses." The answers you'll get will be completely meaningless. Everyone will tell you that they are sometimes too much of a perfectionist or that they're a workaholic. A better way to ask about any potential weaknesses that might give you more meaningful information is,

> How would your best friend describe you?

This question catches most candidates off guard and creates a new, less formal mindset that might force them to drop their guard, potentially allowing you access to information that they would otherwise not have shared.

Have a list of questions that you stick to during any job interview. Use the same questions for all the candidates applying for the same role. Like a research paper, you need to have the same interventions, in this case the questions, because your candidates are all different. You can't have different interventions and different candidates; it will not yield any meaningful results.

References and referees are helpful, but not if you use them in the way that the candidate intends you to use them. Instead, contact them using a technique that no one else will have thought of. If you speak to a referee about the candidate, they have agreed to provide a reference for, you're likely to get excellent feedback that's potentially inaccurate. A better way is to ask your candidate to provide an email address and a phone number for their references. Send a text or an email to all the referees simultaneously. The message should be identical, treat this as a science experiment and reduce the confounders.

The message should have the usual information about why you're contacting them and end with the following novel instructions:

> If your recommendation is less than eight out of ten, please ignore this message.

By adding this ending, you're giving the person who may have reluctantly agreed to be listed as a referee a way out. If challenged, they could say that they didn't get the text or email; it went to spam or a whole host of other plausible excuses. They can't do that if you actually speak to them.

I love to put hurdles in the way of cold candidates. A 'cold candidate' is one who has not been recommended by someone you already know or trust, they might be someone you've found on an online hiring site like Fiverr or Upwork, or someone who has contacted you directly, like a cold caller. These obstacles are an excellent way to test many different qualities you're looking for in an employee or contractor.

One of the best challenges I use is to ask a candidate to complete a task, which could be as simple as their covering letter or application. Once completed, they are instructed to upload the document in a pdf format to a secure cloud folder reserved for applicants to this job. You can choose different tasks depending on what you're trying to test; for example, a task for a receptionist who may be required to work with different file formats and cloud-based servers will not be suitable as a task for a new graduate physiotherapist who is likely to be computer literate.

A suitable task to test a new graduate therapist who will be required to build an exercise video library for your patient base is to send you a thirty-second video about why they're the right person for this job. If the position requires editing post-filming and uploading to your social media channels, that may be the second part of the test.

Always check the social media feeds of any potential candidate. Social media feeds are free for everyone to look at if the account owner makes the content public. This is legitimate research. There is, however, no point in just looking through the feed without purpose or objectives. You need to have defined criteria that you'll use to arrive at concrete decisions. Your defined criteria always relate back to whether the candidate is someone who you think you can work with; they might share similar hobbies, interests, follow the same sporting team for example. The feed can also provide you with useful starting points during an interview; you have mutual friends or you both went to the same university or training college.

The tables can be turned by a candidate. Social media feeds are not only the domain of the business owner. If you're thinking about applying for a job, look at their website and their social media feeds. Ask yourself is this business going to provide me with support, an opportunity to learn from a variety of people with years of experience, a mature mentorship program, an excellent reputation and finally what are their values and beliefs about health and their contribution to their community of patients and clients. If these things resonate with you then you're off to a good start.

Likewise, if you're the business owner, you should be aware that potential therapists can be browsing your site, even if you're not advertising a job. You should always be ready to hire, and you should regularly check the passive advertising on your websites, social media accounts and branding is a true reflection of who you are, how you do things and what you do.

I have used the following questions in many interviews; they are great at extracting important information about the personality, habits, weaknesses, strengths and suitability of a candidate for the role. You should be aiming for the feeling that you get when you're chatting with a person you haven't seen for a while.

How do you alleviate stress?
» Life can be stressful, and every job has some degree of anxiety. So, if someone responds by saying they don't get stressed or claiming not to do anything about it, they are either lying or do not know how to manage it. You should be very interested in how they deal with stress; their answers need to be credible and shouldn't contradict the social media feed research you've conducted.

What are your short-term goals? And long-term goals?
» The response to these questions usually reveals whether the candidate is a thinker and a planner or has more of a laissez-faire attitude. Like all these questions, there's no right or wrong answer. Always look for people who you enjoy talking to.

What type of work environment do you prefer?

» If you have a culture based on mediation, yoga and quiet reflection, don't employ the candidate that likes to work with the sound of AC/DC playing on Spotify. However, if you want to change the existing culture and disrupt the sound environment, then this person might be the outlier you're looking for. Great hires don't have to be like you or clones of your team, just liked by you and your team.

How do you typically deal with conflict?

» This is another question that they will not be expecting. The fall-back answer that most will give is that they will be like His Holiness, the 14th Dalai Lama, in their ability to show compassion, empathy and loving kindness. To find out how they will really react, ask them to give you an example of how they resolved a dispute they had in the last three months.

What do you like to read?

» This loaded question establishes *if* the candidate reads, not *what* they read. If what they read is important to you as an employer, then you should ask them that question specifically. Perhaps one of the roles in this position is that the new team member will be asked to present recent evidence for common MSK conditions to the rest of your staff. If they don't read journals, that might be an issue. You can add a bonus question that asks the candidate what they feel about a recent paper that dismisses a commonly used approach. I would be looking for a demonstration of balance and objective reasoning skills in their answer.

What do you think about the role of manipulation in the treatment of (e.g. chronic lower back pain? or What do you think about the efficacy of (a particular modality, such as RockTape®)?

» We all know there are professional rivalries, within professions and between them. You can exploit this fact by asking these sorts of questions. If you have others in your practice who feel strongly in favour of using a particular treatment, but your candidate feels strongly against it, this might be an interesting talking point, or it might be a concern. Once again, it's not the RockTape® that's the issue; it's how they deal with different professional opinions. Are they going to get on with your team?

What separates you from other therapists or new grads?

» Some candidates have interesting characteristics and experiences that will not be exposed without asking a question like this. Again, the answer to this question helps you to get to know the candidate better and possibly find shared interests, values, habits or experiences. For example, you might find out they volunteered as a trainer for their local sports team or helped patients at the drug and alcohol rehab community centre during their undergraduate training. The answers to these questions, in fact to all interview questions help to create a more relaxed atmosphere and enable you to find out more about the person in front of you.

Tell me how you dealt with the last patient you treated who was worse or just no better after treatment.

» This question applies equally to a recent graduate and an experienced therapist. The recent graduate may have had this experience in the student clinic and the experienced therapist, at their current or previous job.

» You're testing for honesty here. If a candidate is unable to recall a single episode of either of these events, you're talking to a person who either doesn't see many patients, thinks that the patients who don't come back must all be better, never contacts patients who don't come back or is simply suffering from an extreme case of overconfidence bias syndrome.

We covered hiring but we shouldn't forget firing. I've only ever said, "You're fired" once, and I don't regret it. There's no need to go into the reasons why here and obviously not who I said this to. Suffice to say that firing must be the last resort and performed quickly. If you delay your decision, the consequences could be disastrous.

If you ever have to terminate a staff member's employment, never do this without first checking with a lawyer versed in employment law whether it is legal. You may think that you have every reason and right as an employer to end someone's contract, but the law may not agree with you. After you ask someone to leave, the last thing you need is to end up in a messy, painful and expensive legal battle.

If you are an employee or contractor and would like to terminate your employment prematurely, check your rights first. Don't make the appointment with your resignation letter in hand before you know what you are doing is supported by the relevant laws.

Whether you need to terminate a contract or leave a position as the contractor/employee due to disagreement, the meeting between you and the other party must be like a Cold War prisoner exchange scene. Make sure you rehearse the exchange and assume your opponent has done the same; it becomes a formality as you both walk in opposite directions across the bridge. No surprises.

Imaginary rules

YUVAL NOAH HARARI, the acclaimed Israeli author and historian, rightly posits that

> any large-scale human cooperation – whether a modern state, a medieval church, an ancient city, or an archaic tribe – is rooted in common myths that exist only in people's collective imagination.

The legal system is no exception. It is a complex set of imaginary and arbitrary rules designed to control human behaviour and conduct. A legal contract is an example of an agreement between two people or entities. The person who creates the contract has had the contract drawn up for them by a person who interprets the arbitrary rules that society has made up. This person is otherwise known as a 'lawyer'. The person who has commissioned the contract, usually the employer, can be thought of as the player with the white pieces in a game of chess. They have the upper hand because they get to make the first move.

Like a conflict, each side responds to the other's move until finally the battle stops, and a ceasefire is announced. A contract ceasefire is like a war: there are no clear winners; each side has tried to gain the advantage, jostled for control, conceded and gained ground until, finally, a compromise is reached. The final contract is never precisely what both sides wished for.

Contracts are part of our lives, whatever we think about their validity or necessity. Anything that you buy online requires that you, as the buyer, tick the terms and conditions box, confirming that you agree with the contract between you, the purchaser, and the vendor. Buying a house or car, buying an app, undergoing a surgical procedure or hiring a car all require you to sign a contract. They are a part of our litigious society.

As a manual therapist, you will probably have to agree to and sign an employment contract. So, what should you include in your contract as the employer, and what should you expect to be defined in your agreement as the contractor or employee?

The biggest mistake that business owners make when drawing up a contract is that they don't test the arbitrary rules they've included in the agreement. There are many ways to create a contract when employing a healthcare professional. You can download a template online then change the terms and definitions according to your particular circumstances. You can ask a lawyer to draft a contract for you, which they will base on a similar one that they've already created as a template for your profession in general. Or you could just create your own from scratch. Whichever of these choices you make about the source of your contract, you must test the rules that you set out before you agree upon them with the other party. It's a bit like researching the best way to make a cake, spending hours putting it together, then finally marvelling at the masterpiece before your eyes, only to find that someone's allergic to nuts!

One of the best ways to test your contract is to have it audited by the very people that will scrutinise the agreement in the case of a dispute. The most appropriate auditors are the government bodies that will adjudicate in favour of the employer, the worker or the contractor once a challenge is lodged. Contract inclusions can be tested online using government websites. The Australian Taxation Office has a convenient online tool called an Employee/Contractor decision tool. It can be used to help determine whether a worker is an employee or contractor for tax and superannuation purposes.

The beauty of testing a contract is that it gives you leverage. Once you test the contract, it becomes a valuable document that you can use repeatedly. This saves you time, money and reduces the possibility of a successful legal challenge. The more time you spend on creating a fair, respectful and transparent workplace contract, the more likely you will be able to use it time and time again without challenge.

Many therapists are employed as contractors or associates within a group practice. The definition of a contractor is often misunderstood because it's a grey area of the law. At the time of writing, a contractor in Australia is generally independent of the employer.

Essentially, a contractor is operating their own business within another business using their own equipment, working for more than one employer, choosing their own times of work, responsible for their own insurance, and making their own decisions about their fees.

The more you veer from these principles in your contract, the more likely it is that Health and Safety regulators, taxation offices and insurers will deem your contract to be on the greyer end of the scale and, as such, deem your agreement is one between an employer and a worker, not a contractor.

TAKE ACTION

Avoid confusion, stress, unexpected financial liability and a legal challenge by checking your employment contract, and make sure the answers to the questions listed below are crystal clear, whether you are the employer, contractor or employee.

Questions for Employers

- » Who is your contract with? An employee or a contractor?
- » Who is responsible for the treatment of the clinic's patients?
- » Whose name is on the clinic's invoice? The contractor's or the employer's?
- » What will your clinic provide the contractor or employee? (e.g. linen, a treatment room, a treatment bed, reception cover)
- » Who is responsible for promoting the services you offer?
- » Who is liable should the contractor or employee become injured, sick or unable to work?

Questions for contractors and employees

- » Who is responsible for paying for my superannuation?
- » Who is responsible for paying my tax?
- » How often will I get the money I receive from patients?
- » Who is responsible for reconciling the payments I receive from patients?

- » Who is responsible for paying my registration fee?
- » Who is responsible for paying my Public Liability & Professional Indemnity Insurance?
- » As a contractor, should I have to indemnify the clinic resulting from harm or loss related to the provision of my services?
- » What is my management fee and how is it paid to the practice owner?
- » When will the management fee be reviewed, and which metrics will be used to determine change?
- » Will I be asked to achieve specific KPIs?
- » What is the required notice period?
- » Will I be required to perform any other duties such as PD sessions or advertising/marketing?
- » Who receives the money that patients or clients pay for their treatment?
- » Who decides on the hours of my work?

"The best yes is to say no"

GREG McKEOWN, the British author of the *New York Times* and *Wall Street Journal* bestseller, *Essentialism: The Disciplined Pursuit of Less* (2014) is in high demand as a public speaker and regularly presents to companies like LinkedIn, Google, Facebook, Apple, Pixar and Twitter. The first time I read his book was two years after I launched CPD Health Courses, an education business for health professionals. My wife and I started this business, having seen a niche in the market. There were only three companies that were teaching dry needling in Australia at the time.

I saw an opportunity in how courses were delivered to time-poor health professionals. Educators were still using boring PowerPoint slides to teach the prerequisite theory, wasting valuable time and money. None of them used the available technologies to present the theory online despite the worldwide trend towards this inevitable platform. To this day, no one is truly able to compete with our state of the art, custom-built software that allows healthcare professionals who want to learn dry needling skills to complete their online theory in their own time on any device connected to the internet.

Before we advertised our first course in our hometown of Melbourne, Australia, we planned to present four courses a year, one in each state in the country. I remember asking our programmer to launch our website to the world in January 2013. We were enjoying a family holiday in Queensland with our three children. The response was literally like releasing tickets to a Katie Perry concert. Our first course was sold out in minutes. In fact, we had to schedule a second course on the following weekend to accommodate the excess interest. During the first few minutes of watching the enrolments come in, I knew we had created something meaningful and valuable; we had disrupted the existing market.

Since our first two courses in Melbourne, things have snowballed, and we are now the largest provider of dry needling education in

Australia. We present over sixty-six courses in five capital cities throughout Australia. Despite the many time challenges that I encountered during those early years, I found time to read Greg McKeown's book a second time – I always read great books twice. I got so much more after reading this seminal work a second time. The one thing that stuck in my mind is Greg's quote, "the best yes is to say no". This powerful statement can change how we think and respond to the demands of our professional lives and our daily personal challenges.

At every opportunity, I have used Greg's advice and thought about the concepts that he clearly presents in his book. I must be honest, I do lapse from time to time, but in general, without this information, I would have been pulled in so many directions that I would have become highly ineffective, never having achieved the many milestones we've accomplished in our education business.

McKeown is not saying that we need to say no to every demand presented to us, but to be much more discerning about our choices when we accept new projects, employment, hours of work, helping others or further study. Sometimes, when reading a book with such a strong message, it's very easy to walk away with the false assumption that all one has to do is say no to everything. However, by inference, saying no to one thing is saying yes to something else. If you say no to social media distractions while you're reading an important book, you are saying yes to immersing yourself in the book and fully investing in a learning journey. If you say no to all calls while you're treating patients, you're saying yes to being present and deliberate about everything you're doing in your treatment room.

Suppose you say no to extending your opening hours to accommodate patients who work late. In that case, you are saying yes to staying true to the patients you want to attract and serve rather than trying to be everything to everybody, which inevitably results in your business being nothing to anyone.

A classic work–life balance question when you're building a business, a brand or your experience is the time you spend working versus the time you spend with family and friends. I can think of many occasions when I decided to add another patient to my full list when I should have said no. It's not easy to do this, but I learnt that it was much harder to undo the damage that saying yes was doing to my energy levels, concentration and ability to engage with the most important people in my life.

I still remember to this day, a conversation that I had while I was treating my last patient one Saturday. My receptionist had gone home because I had added him at the end of my full Saturday morning list. He was the last client of the day. I finished treating him and met him at the front desk. I had no back up, just him and me at the reception desk looking at my full list on the following Saturday. Naturally, the patient wanted another appointment at a time convenient for him. It turned out that he found this appointment time very convenient and wanted another one, at the same time, next week.

Of course, he didn't know that I had just finished the chapter in Greg's book in which he explains how he managed the inevitable distractions while trying to write his book. Greg uses a term that stuck in my mind: he went into monk mode – no email, no phone, no Google, no social media, and a blank screen to write on. I used the advice that Greg gave in this chapter to create my own strategy for managing this recurring challenge, which I have always found difficult to handle. My answer, like all natural and sensible responses, was the truth. When asked if I could add another appointment to my list next Saturday, I said no. But you can't just say, no. You must give the why. That's where the absolute honesty begins. I added this sentence to the no: "I'm sorry, but I can't see you at that time next week because that's my family time. I hope that's okay."

In almost every situation, whether your boss asks you to stay later and see an emergency patient, act as the clinic professional development coordinator or wait for your pay rise until next year, the correct and only answer is no, followed by the honest why.

Borrowing from others

ONE OF THE MOST IMPORTANT QUESTIONS that you need to answer, whether you employ others in a healthcare business, work in a healthcare business as a contractor or employee, or work on your own, is 'why?'. Your 'why' is your value proposition (VP).

I had been thinking about our education business, CPD Health Courses' VP for months, the reason customers would choose us over and above any other education business. What was our 'why'? What was that reason? What made us different? What made us special or unique?

The answer was powerful and impactful. It would impact every business decision that we would make in the future, and if I looked back on our past choices, I would clearly see how it had already influenced those I had made in the past. Like all great solutions, it would be like the last piece in a jigsaw, which finally completes the 'why' picture about us. That final piece adds significant meaning to what was previously incomplete and unclear to our prospects.

Creating a value proposition shifts you from the unenviable position of being something to everyone and inevitably failing because that common business strategy results in being nothing to anyone. Once created, our company 'why' would elevate us into the rarefied air, shared with only those businesses that choose to be everything to a few. Our VP would provide us with great confidence in our future decision-making and strategies because of the solid foundations that our 'why' was built on. It would not just influence our decisions, but new ideas and solutions that evolved from them.

Over the years, I had learnt that trying to force an answer seldom works. If I have many possible answers going around my mind, they are all competing with each other, trying to be the one reason 'why', it means that I haven't reached the required still point of rare clarity. I would know when I had reached this point, and I knew that the solution would be worth waiting for. My answer had to be one that couldn't be challenged by further thinking or doubts that naturally occur after making a final decision as necessary as this – no other reason why it would be better, even though my monkey mind would do its best to try and topple the winner off the podium.

All industries and professions have unique challenges, including the healthcare professions, but I have found that the best solutions to these challenges can be found outside the respective profession. I have borrowed ideas from the aviation industry, online shopping giants, courier companies, the legal profession and the food industry. I cannot think of the last idea or solution that I found within health care that solved a problem or challenge that I was presented with.

On the day I found the last jigsaw piece which created our company's value proposition, I was sitting on a Qantas flight. It was soon after a period of rapid growth in our business and great excitement. While seated on the flight and waiting for the doors to shut, a single word popped into my mind. That word became our value proposition and the primer to the tag line in all our subsequent branding, marketing and advertising. 'Safety' had become our VP. The jigsaw piece was such a good fit that we trademarked the combination together with two other words: Safe. Confident. Effective.

The aviation industry's inherent framework had provided my subconscious mind with the term 'safety'. Everything about the experience of flying was built on this potent and arresting word. It is critical to understand and follow safety when travelling by plane – starting from the baggage check-in questions about what is in your luggage and who did the packing, to the security screening, the signage in an airport and on board, the language used by the crew and ground staff, the emergency demonstration and the safety instructions printed in the pocket of every seat. Aviation was entirely analogous for presenting dry needling courses in so many ways.

When you find your value proposition, great things happen. Adding anything to it makes both look better. Like the marquee player in a football team, he looks great on his own, but the rest of his teammates suddenly shine too. Safety was now our raison d'être. It became the thread that weaves its way through everything we do and say in all our communication.

Manual therapists do business with CPD Health Courses because they will leave our courses feeling that they can safely practise dry needling, unburdened by a single doubt about causing harm to their patients or reputations. They choose us over any of our competitors because they see, hear and read that safety is embedded in everything we do, and we communicate that to the manual therapists who are our customers. Therapists who complete our training will report that the single most important reason why they chose us was our commitment and attention to safety.

Since creating our VP of safety, our data shows that 93 per cent of all our customers stated that safety was the primary reason they chose CPD Health Courses to complete their dry needling training. Week in, week out, the answer to the question on our evaluation form, "Why did you choose CPD Health Courses?", safety is listed as the main reason. This is compelling reading for any business owner.

The other two words, 'confident' and 'effective', came very quickly after deciding on safety as the first word in our tagline because it was the right marquee word. When you complete our dry needling training, you will feel *safe*. That is a fact, but what then? Safe is the only status we will guarantee. Beyond this, we cannot promise any other feelings, attributes or accolades for the manual therapists who successfully complete our dry needling courses.

Confidence is a state that will develop over time, just like effectiveness. You cannot be confident about all the skills you have learnt in our courses. You could be confident about a few techniques but not so much about some of the others. Likewise, you cannot, therefore, be effective in delivering all the new techniques you will learn. This only happens with experience. Given that confidence and effectiveness are not guaranteed, they follow safety in a specific order rather than lead our tagline.

> **TAKE ACTION**
>
> What is your value proposition? To answer this critical question, you need to start with your 'why?'. To help you get started, I recommend that you watch the TED Talk by Simon Sinek, author of the book, *Start With Why*. Then ask yourself the following questions:

Why do you do what you do?

» No, the answers can't be ... because it'll give me a good income, you love working for yourself or because you really like people. These answers are too vague. You need to search deep inside yourself for a solution that doesn't involve you. If you come up with an answer and then start thinking, but everyone says that. That will be because everyone does say that. Your answer needs to be specific, targeted, unique and exclusive to you or your company.

What are you most passionate about when it comes to your work?

» This could be a technique that you've mastered or developed or it could be great success that you've had treating a particular condition, or a subgroup of patients that you have attracted. The word 'passionate' is overused these days; you will know if you are passionate about anything if you start to get a lump in your throat talking about it. The sort of throat discomfort you feel when talking about a loved one or something that means everything to you. If you don't feel it, you're not passionate about it. You just think you should be.

» A few years ago, I recorded a short video to promote my Dry Needling Video Training membership site. This is another part of our education business that helps therapists refresh and review their dry needling skills. The all-day event involved the videographer and marketing specialist I engaged asking me a question, which I would answer while looking directly into the camera lens. When he asked me a simple and quite reasonable question, "Why should someone join my membership site?" I started to feel a lump in my throat. I knew that what I said was from my heart, it was honest, raw and real. I spoke about my obsession with safety and wanting to raise the standards of dry needling education with clarity and deep emotion. I said that my goal was to help create future generations of the safest dry needling therapists in the world, and I meant it. All this was possible because I was already clear about the why in my business.

If you imagine yourself as your ideal customer, would your offer be enough to differentiate you from your competitors? Would you choose yourself as the winner?

» If not, then that won't work. The acid test for any service industry professional is to put themselves in their customer's shoes. Answer the question that your intended target market might ask, "Why A over B?" Unless you can, hand on heart, say that your offer leaves B for dead, it isn't enough.

» Suppose I audited everything about my business, including my language, behaviour, website, branding, advertising, team, signage and communication. Would my ideal customer be able to arrive at my value proposition on their own? If not, then you don't have your VP yet.

How much are you worth?

PABLO RUIZ PICASSO was born in Malaga, Spain in 1881. He became one of the most influential artists of the 20th century. His legacy lives on in many of the creative fields. In addition to being a master painter, he was a sculptor, ceramicist, printmaker and stage designer.

Picasso's mother, Maria Picasso López, claimed that his first word was not *mamá* but *piz*, a shortened version of '*lápiz*', which means pencil in Spanish. He was destined for great things from an early age. His first teacher was his father, José Ruiz Blasco, a professor of drawing. As is common in many, if not all, father–son relationships, Picasso quickly surpassed his father's talents and hosted his first exhibition at age thirteen in *A Coruña*.

His artistic career continued to flourish while he was living in Barcelona and Madrid until 1904 when he moved to France, where he lived for the rest of his life.

Picasso is perhaps best known for pioneering Cubism, a revolutionary modern artistic style that depicted objects from multiple views on a single canvas, creating illusions and new perspectives. Picasso is not only one of history's most famous artists, but his painting *Guernica* which depicts the town during the Spanish Civil War in 1937, is one of the most online searched-for painting titles in the world. Picasso died in Mougins, France, in 1973 at the age of ninety after a career that spanned almost eighty years, leaving behind more than 50,000 artworks, including paintings, drawings, sculpture, ceramics and prints.

There are many versions of this famous but possibly apocryphal story about Picasso; it involves a coffee shop, a fan and a napkin. The stories are slightly different in their settings, but the take-home message is consistent.

One day, Picasso is sitting in a French coffee shop, casually doodling on a white napkin with his familiar charcoal pencil. One of his most fervent admirers sat across the room, watching the Spanish master with increasing interest. A few minutes later, Picasso stops sketching, rises from his chair, folds the napkin into his jacket pocket and starts making his way towards the door. Recognising this rare opportunity, the art lover walks over to Picasso and politely asks him if she can buy the napkin, he had just drawn on. Picasso says, "Yes, of course, it will cost you 100,000 francs."

Shocked at the price of a simple drawing on a coffee shop napkin, the woman says, "but I watched you draw. It took you no longer than four or five minutes." Picasso replies with his incisive answer:

> It didn't take me four or five minutes; it took me a lifetime.

The take-home message is that Picasso's artistic works are indexed to his experience and knowledge.

As a manual therapist, the value of your treatment five years from now will be, or perhaps more accurately *should be*, more valuable than those that you deliver today. That's because your experience, technical ability, pattern recognition and knowledge will all increase over time, assuming you continue to learn. Your experience at the time of any particular treatment is the culmination of everything you know at that time. These are essential considerations for setting your professional fees and the equally important decisions about incremental increases over time.

I have always believed that the professional fees in a large group clinic with a range of experience levels should reflect the differences in service levels rather than a socialist pricing approach. Scaling your fee structure allows your customers to select based on an additional variable; this can be advantageous for those who have not been referred to a particular therapist at your clinic and can freely choose solely based on price.

A range of fees commensurate with experience levels enables a broader appeal to your prospects at either end of the spectrum. Don't be surprised if patients choose a therapist based on nothing other than the fact they have the highest fees. The fees must represent the real and tangible benefits for a patient and not abstract criteria that bear no direct relationship to value and service. Just because a therapist is a course junky, attending and completing more weekend postgraduate training than any of their colleagues, does not mean that their fees should be greater than the therapist who is too busy to attend courses because their list is always full.

Experience is not the sole driver of fees. Many therapists have been in practice for several decades, but they are still struggling to fill their list or retain patients. The one indisputable factor that should always take centre stage when deciding on fees is 'bums on seats' created by the age-old fundamental relationship between supply and demand. If you have a full list, you need to consider increasing your prices.

Setting your professional fees can be difficult. There are so many factors to consider, including your demographic, your professional experience, practice overheads, competitor fees, recommendations by your professional association and how much your colleagues charge within the practice you work.

I have found a much simpler way to ensure that you've set your fees at the right level. Of course, there are essential considerations that need to be factored in, but in the end, the best way to make sure you've considered all the variables correctly is a subjective one that relies on gut feeling.

If you work in a clinic that employs a receptionist, you will have been shielded from the crude and dirty business of asking and accepting money from your patients or clients. This arrangement has inoculated us against the sometimes uncomfortable feelings associated with valuing our services. The use of a phone or a credit card to pay for professional fees has also made the financial transaction at the end of a treatment a little more abstract rather than the handling of real money in the form of notes and even coins.

To determine if you have set your fees at the right level, imagine yourself without the protection of a receptionist and ask yourself if you would feel comfortable directly asking your patient for the amount you are asking for in return for your services. If you have set your fees too high, you may feel that you are getting away with the amount you're asking for, and you feel a little embarrassed about charging too high a fee.

If you've set your fees too low, you'll feel that you've given away too much, and your patients are getting a real bargain. If you've set your fees at the right level, you'll feel comfortable and confident when asking for your fee, knowing that it represents equal value for what you've provided.

Set and forget

I REMEMBER COMING HOME after another exhausting week in the clinic during the winter of 2008. At the time, I was treating sixty to seventy patients a week. I would finish at 1 pm on Saturday, come home and slump in front of the TV, not wanting to talk to another living soul for at least twenty-four hours. One such Saturday afternoon, I stumbled across an interview with Mike O'Hagan, owner of the removalist company, Mini Movers, on the Sky Business Channel.

From my semi-comatose state, I sprung to life as I heard what he said about running a successful business. In the brief segment about successful entrepreneurship, Mike described how he had built his business empire, which now turns over twenty-three million dollars annually. He pinpointed all the pain points I was experiencing as if he could read my tired mind.

It was as if he was speaking to me in my lounge room rather than through the TV speakers. I was so taken aback by his story that I immediately found a way to contact him, and to my surprise, he agreed to meet up a few days later. It only took me a few minutes with Mike to realise what an opportunity I had before me at our first meeting. I asked Mike to mentor me, to which he agreed. I learnt so much from him. He had the ability to get straight to the point. It was as if the tables were turned and he was the therapist taking a case history for my presenting complaint. He asked the right questions, which made efficient use of our meeting time.

Like a detective, he had a way of parsing the information given to him and systematically working through a mental flowchart to arrive at the crux of my problem. Once a challenge was identified, the solution was swiftly and clearly presented. The best thing about our mentoring meetings is that Mike had nothing to do with health care, so he always tried to be unbiased and untainted when offering advice.

The first piece of advice I got from him was to buy a book called, *The E-Myth: Why Most Businesses Don't Work and What to Do About It*, written by American Michael E. Gerber (2012). The E in the E-Myth book title stands for 'entrepreneurial'.

Inc. Magazine calls Gerber "the World's #1 Small Business Guru" – the entrepreneurial and small-business thought leader who has impacted the lives of millions of small-business owners and hundreds of thousands of companies worldwide for over forty years.

Since writing his first bestseller in 1986, Gerber later wrote an updated and revised edition in 1995 dispelling the myths about starting one's own business. He has since written nineteen additional books especially for specific professions and industries, including lawyers, accountants, optometrists, chiropractors, landscape contractors, financial advisers, architects, real estate brokers, insurance agents, dentists, nutritionists, bookkeepers, veterinarians, real estate investors, real estate agents and chief financial officers. Gerber's mission is trademarked: "to transform the state of small business worldwide™".

Once I started reading *The E-Myth*, I could see why Mike had recommended it to me. Gerber's guide about how to build a turnkey business that didn't need you was precisely what Mini-Movers turned out to be.

Mike started in business as a second-hand dealer at the age of twenty-eight. The company grew, and soon he was working ninety hours a week but earning less than his employees, who were all working forty hours a week. Using duplication and systemisation to leverage everything he did, Mike switched his managerial mindset to entrepreneurship, which allowed him to exit the business but retain full family ownership. Leaving the company allowed Mike to finally work *on* his business rather than *in* it.

There are usually only one or two events in one's life that truly change your course. In my case, reading *The E-Myth* in 2008 was pivotal in my business life. I started to wake up and search for answers and solutions to the daily challenges of business ownership. I couldn't put the book down. I listened to the audio version six times in the space of a month and asked my wife to read it simultaneously, so we could discuss what we had learnt. I played it when I was in the car, at the gym, instead of watching television at night, and between patients.

The E-Myth is based on the story of Sarah, a passionate, hardworking woman and business owner who loved to bake pies. She opened a bakery and started to work until, eventually, the hard work turned her love for pies into hate. The reality of running a business, hiring staff, working long hours, waking up early every day, and making almost no money after all the expenses were paid lead to burnout; that is, until she decides to apply the advice from her mentor, Michael Gerber, who turns things around by using the principles he explains in his book. I was so inspired by the book that I immediately engaged an E-Myth business coach to help me apply the recommended principles discussed in the book.

The E-Myth premise is that you cannot successfully operate any business if it relies solely on you. Whether you're a contractor or a healthcare business owner, you must implement systems and strategies that remove the dependence on your physical work. I realised that I was a great technician, just like many manual therapists. I knew how to do my job, and I did it very well. This, however, did not mean that I knew how to run a business. Technical knowhow doesn't mean business expertise; far from it, in fact. Gerber explains why everyone who goes into business needs to divide their work into three parts: technician, manager and entrepreneur.

My work life was heavily skewed towards the physical work of treating patients, and I wasn't paying attention to the equally important roles of being creative and developing ideas as an entrepreneur or the setting up of systems and workflows that a manager must put in place for everyone employed in my business. The take-home lesson that I learnt from Mike O'Hagan and *The E-Myth* was to set and forget everything, every time. Once you learn to set and forget the most critical tasks in your business, you can leverage the work you've put in to gain passive returns, over and over again, just like a passive income.

Leverage is the most effective tool I have at my disposal now. I try to use it to maximise my returns on all my daily tasks. I put the hard work in early, with an eye on never having to do the same job more than once. This 'set and forget' habit has paid huge dividends for me, not only in business but in my home and personal life.

Everyone can use the set and forget mentality; like every habit, you just have to ask yourself,

> How can I complete this task once and reap the rewards on multiple occasions in the future?

There are many examples of this in everyday practice, including developing a comprehensive, transparent, honest and fair contract between you and your staff. Consult your team, pay for legal advice, make the final changes, test it, and then use it repeatedly.

Create your social media checklist, decide who is responsible for each task and decide when and how often each task must be completed. List the order in which each step must be completed. Assign someone other than you to manage the job and walk away. Stand back and marvel at how the social media machine churns out consistent results without your input. When I say walk away, I am referring to you as the employer who delegates a task to someone other than you or indeed the delegate themselves. If you are delegated a task that does not mean that you need to complete everything that is part of that task yourself, after consultation, you may have to delegate some of these tasks to others more qualified or skilled.

Find the busiest person in your therapist team. Give them the job of organising the professional development calendar for your clinic. Give them direction about content, duration, presenter fees and presentation frequency. Set up a time to meet again, then see what they come up with. Your calendar will be complete in a short period of time, filled with regular presenters who provide excellent content fulfilling your staff PD requirements.

My 'set and forget' mentality gives me more time, time to be creative in my business planning and ideas. I have time to think about what will make the most significant differences and provide our customers and our staff with tremendous gains. I no longer live in the thick weeds of management, but rather, I search for the highest vantage points, from where I can observe and make better decisions that will lead to better outcomes.

> **TAKE ACTION**
>
> List all the tasks that you perform over the next month. Review the way that you complete each task.
>
> **Ask yourself ...**

- Can I save time and money by doing this task differently?
- Can anyone other than me complete this task quicker, better, more efficiently or more cheaply?
- What are the roadblocks that stop me from setting and forgetting this task?
- Am I micromanaging any of these tasks and subsequently preventing others who may be more qualified than I am from accessing this task?
- Am I denying someone in my team valuable experience and practice opportunities by giving someone a fish rather than teaching them how to fish?
- What are the recurring tasks that require the same processes?
- How much time do I want to spend on each task?
- Is there any technology out there that can complete some of these tasks more quickly?

What next?

WELL, THAT WAS THE EASY BIT. Reading is enjoyable and requires minimal effort on the part of the reader. Doing is much more challenging.

Let's suppose that you're going to make some changes to the way you operate your business after reading this book. You might decide to change the way you onboard your new patients, tweak your website, create front desk scripts, set up an automated GP referral letter, start journaling, develop an undergraduate training program, or find a business mentor when you're ready. You might not be ready right now.

> When the student is ready, the teacher will appear. When the student is truly ready, the teacher will disappear.

The origin of this quote is contested. Some attribute it to Buddha Siddhartha Gautama Shakyamuni; others cite a more recent theosophical source dating back to the late 1800s. In the end, it doesn't really matter who said this first; what matters are the words themselves. We should not allow the intellectual debate to distract us from the true value of the quote's meaning. I think that the quote is entirely valid and accurately reflects my earlier learning experiences. Once I finish a book that offers advice and a new perspective, or challenges my existing thought processes, I don't always spring into action and make immediate changes to my life or business. I need to be in the right frame of mind to work on meaningful change. This is not a cop-out or laziness on my part; I'm just honest. If I've ever tried to push through because I feel guilty that I've spent time reading, listening, or attending a course but haven't acted upon it, I am guaranteed to fail.

Exposure to new information, whether through books, audio or face-to-face courses, sometimes leads to learning and learning sometimes leads to change. If you're not ready, you'll slide down the process very quickly and end up further back than where you started due to the disappointment of failure. Then you'll need even more enthusiasm than you artificially mustered in the first place to get back to the start line.

No one should change anything because someone tells them to. It must come from within that person because they want or need to change. People wrongly think that all you need to do is just get on with it. I disagree. The 'just getting on with it' approach never works. There must be a compelling reason for starting a new task or project or making changes. The reason might be that something in your business isn't working well, making it harder for your team or you to deliver your product or service. Once you recognise and accept that there's a problem, you have to decide whether it's worth your time to do anything about it. Not every issue has to be fixed. It depends on the impact that problem is having on your business.

My process for deciding whether to act or delay involves actively placing a series of mental hurdles in the way of my thinking processes. If an idea or change manages to get past my intentional mental hurdles, it deserves to be acted upon. It's my way of ensuring that the reason for implementing change is clear and beyond challenge.

All change worthy of action requires a degree of mental stamina to get the job done and sometimes defend one's decision to others. Your decision to change the way you do things may affect only a few people or it may affect many people. In general, people don't like change. This is well recognised in the corporate world. Large corporates have highly trained professionals, called 'change management experts', to help teams accept and work with new software, procedures, systems, equipment or even mindsets.

Working in this way enables clarity of thought along the way and unparalleled efficiency of thought. Because the mental hurdles are now behind you, you only have eyes on the prize. There's no extra thinking about the merits of your new journey. If you've got this process right, you shouldn't even have to think, let alone expend energy on extra thinking. The hard work has already been completed. Now you can just get on with it, with vigour, excitement and drive.

If you're ready now, then as I've mentioned before, start at the end. What do you want this to look like when it's finished? The 'this' is your career, contribution, influence, impact, legacy or experience. Once you are clear, begin the doing process.

The most significant gains I have had are from the books that I've read or listened to more than once. I always find that I've missed something or gain new insight the second and even third time around. I could not have written this book without the help of many people. Information is freely and readily available to everyone who has access to the internet. No longer do you have to wait for the library to open on Monday after school, then wait for the librarian to tell you that the book you want is on the shelves or on loan.

Decide if you want to know more about anything you've read in this book. If you need help, find a mentor who can help you with your business, technical skills, marketing, advertising, social media, web development or any other aspect of your professional skill set. The section 'Teachers, mentors and resilience' might be a good place to start.

I hope that my book has achieved the one thing that I set out to do: to help you realise how fortunate you are to have chosen a career rooted in the belief that you can help someone just using your two hands. I am proud to be part of a profession that combines the art of palpation with an equal measure of continuing scientific knowledge and research.

Dedication

They say that everyone has one book in them. In late 2018, my education business was growing quickly, and my good friend and colleague, Dian Parry, bought me a copy of the book *Key Person of Influence: The Five-Step Method to Become One of the Most Highly Valued and Highly Paid People in Your Industry*, by Daniel Priestley. He told me that I needed to tell my story and write my book. He was right. I had a story to tell but what I didn't know was who the story was for.

Just like all things that feel right, I now know who this book is for. My book is for my daughter, Amina, and everyone like her. Amina is our middle child and in her final year of Osteopathy. When she told me that she is required to complete an internship with an osteopath in private practice as part of her training, I knew what I had to do. I left the clinic that I once owned to start a home-based practice, where it all began twenty-seven years ago. I intend to mentor and support her for the next twelve months until she graduates. I'll teach her everything I know and, like every parent, hope that she eclipses my career.

About the author

DR WAEL MAHMOUD, D.O.,
MAppSci (Acupuncture)
Osteopath & Acupuncturist

Since graduating from the British School of Osteopathy, London, in 1985, I have worked in the healthcare profession as an osteopath and, since 2000, as an acupuncturist. Every time I walk into my treatment room, I still feel the sense of privilege, excitement and honour that I experienced treating my first patient as a new grad, knowing that I have complete autonomy over what I can do to help someone overcome pain, restore function and return to doing what they love.

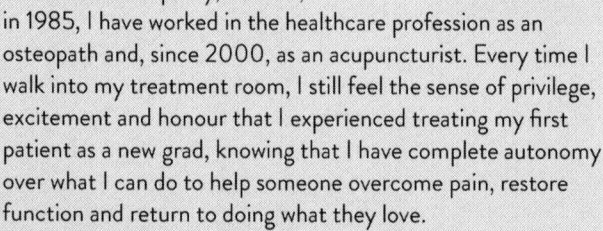

I have a duty to share my knowledge with you because I know that my contribution will help you fulfil your role and responsibility in helping others as a manual therapist, using just your two hands. Those you help will, in turn, be able to help others in their network and community.

I have been very fortunate to have worked as a university lecturer, an associate, locum, employee, contractor and business owner in Australia and the United Kingdom during my career. My experiences have provided a unique perspective for helping manual therapists who work for themselves, employ others or are employees.

Manufactured by Amazon.com.au
Sydney, New South Wales, Australia